PLEASURE IN BIRTH

Pleasure in Birth: Wellbeing, Praxis, and Reproductive Justice explores how birthing people experience pleasure in childbirth, challenging dominant narratives that equate birth solely with pain and suffering.

Drawing on The Birth Pleasure Study—the first rigorous mixed-methods research of its kind—this book presents rich data from 23 interviews covering 43 birth experiences across diverse racial, ethnic, gender, and socio-economic backgrounds. The book weaves experiential accounts with critical analysis to examine how cultural beliefs shape birth experiences and reinforce the maternal health crisis, particularly in the US. By introducing the Pleasure-Forward Birth Model, the book reimagines childbirth as a site of possibility, resilience, and joy, pushing back against the hyper-medicalized and fear-driven status quo.

Pleasure in Birth: Wellbeing, Praxis, and Reproductive Justice is ideal for advanced undergraduates, graduate students, and professional birth workers in the social and medical sciences, especially those interested in reproductive justice, maternal health, and cultural approaches to childbirth.

Elisabeth Bolaza is a critical sexualities scholar, reproductive anthropologist, and maternal health researcher. She is the founder and lead of SORADA, a research consulting practice transforming maternal, sexual, and reproductive health through research, rigor, and praxis. She is based in Oakland, California.

Social Science Perspectives on Childbirth and Reproduction

Series editor:
Robbie Davis-Floyd, Rice University, Houston, Texas

This series focuses on issues relating to childbirth and reproduction from social science perspectives. It includes single-authored, co-authored, or edited books concerned both with people's reproductive experiences and with birth practitioners such as midwives (both professional and traditional), obstetricians, nurses, doulas, and others. It seeks to provide new viewpoints on functional and sustainable birth models and the challenges to their creation and maintenance, as well as on obstetric violence, disrespect, and abuse and their root causes. Single-case or comparative ethnographies on birth and other reproductive issues are featured, from high-tech conceptions to normal pregnancy and birth, including reproductive politics and human-rights issues in reproduction worldwide.

Eggonomics
The Global Market in Human Eggs and the Donors Who Supply Them
Diane M. Tober

Traditional Midwives
Cross-Cultural Perspectives
Edited by Robbie Davis-Floyd, Betty-Anne Daviss and Inayat Ali

Pleasure in Birth
Wellbeing, Praxis, and Reproductive Justice
Elisabeth Bolaza

For more information about this series, please visit: www.routledge.com/Social-Science-Perspectives-on-Childbirth-and-Reproduction/book-series/SSPCR

PLEASURE IN BIRTH

Wellbeing, Praxis, and Reproductive Justice

Elisabeth Bolaza

Routledge
Taylor & Francis Group
NEW YORK AND LONDON

Designed cover image: FatCamera, Getty Images

First published 2026
by Routledge
605 Third Avenue, New York, NY 10158

and by Routledge
4 Park Square, Milton Park, Abingdon, Oxon, OX14 4RN

Routledge is an imprint of the Taylor & Francis Group, an informa business

ISBN: 978-1-032-81366-0 (hbk)
ISBN: 978-1-032-80494-1 (pbk)
ISBN: 978-1-003-49942-8 (ebk)

DOI: 10.4324/9781003499428

Typeset in Sabon
by Newgen Publishing UK

CONTENTS

ACKNOWLEDGEMENTS

First, I want to acknowledge the wise ones, the women, mothers, birth-givers, birth-keepers, healers, midwives, doulas, educators, and scholars. Thank you for bravely preserving these deep rivers of knowledge—against such odds.

I am overwhelmed with gratitude to the many birthing people who raised their hands and voices to co-create this research. Thank you for trusting me with your experiences and with the process of coalescing your wisdom into forms to be shared with others. I am honored beyond measure.

Thank you, Dr. Michelle Marzullo, for chairing my dissertation committee, for empowering me in this unconventional work, and for your bold leadership in the field of Critical Sexuality Studies. Thank you, Dr. Dána-Ain Davis and Dr. Robbie Davis-Floyd for trailblazing this field of reproductive anthropology, and for taking me on as a doctoral student. I am also so grateful to Dr. Robbie Davis-Floyd for inviting me to contribute this research to her curated series, and to Dr. Meagan Simpson, the editor of this book. Thank you for your level-headed guidance, kindness, and support. As a first-generation scholar, I couldn't have wished for a better team. I also owe this book to many teachers who have shaped me over the years. From my sensei Grand Master Frank Daniels (who passed on before this book could be published) to my many professors at UCLA, UC Berkeley's School of Public Health, and the California Institute of Integral Studies, thank you for sparking in me many transformations. Thank you also to Dr. Barbara Katz Rothman, Dr. Monica McLemore, Dr. Karen Scott, Dr. Grace Howard, Debra Pascali Bonaro, and so many others who have shown me what it means to co-conspire for the birth of a better world.

Many people sustained me through the simultaneous adventures of doctoral education, pregnancy, birth and early parenthood of two young children, a global pandemic, and the subsequent and ongoing onslaught of multipronged sociopolitical turmoil. Lynn Wilson, April Berger, Kristine Thompson, Nicole Rangel, Jessamyn Meyerhoff, Renata Moreira, Samsarah Morgan, Oloya Tyehimba-Ford, Meghan Lewis, and also, all the beloved baristas who kept me caffeinated; this work would have been impossible without you.

Now, for my family. Thank you, Mom, for life itself. Grandma Lillyan, you've inspired me and my work more than you know. Thank you for the curiosity you fueled in me, your passionate spirit, and tireless love. Christopher, love of my life, thank you for being my dauntless champion. Lyla and Naomi, my precious children, thank you for the worlds you open for me every day. Thank you for the gifts you are, your dandelion wishes, special rocks, pretty leaves, songs, stories, and all the cute aggression. I love you, forever and ever, no matter what.

INTRODUCTION

Marion's waters suddenly broke two months before her due date. She'd been healthy: a 21-year-old, heterosexual, White woman in her first pregnancy with no major complications. Marion was urgently transported to the nearest hospital facility with a NICU (neonatal intensive care unit). The closest such facility was over an hour's drive from her midwestern rural home in the US. Her partner was unable to go with her because of his work responsibilities. Alone, Marion was kept confined to bedrest for nine grueling days in this hospital. During this time, her care team checked her cervical dilation manually several times, with no discussion of the associated risks. She then developed a serious uterine infection and underwent an emergency cesarean under general anesthesia. Marion awoke over an hour after this procedure and was then informed that a baby girl had been delivered and then transferred to the NICU. Both were hospitalized in intensive care for their serious infections. Marion described through her tears the aftermath of alienation that she'd felt from her own baby and also from herself:

> I just cried and cried and cried for months. … I didn't feel like I'd become a mother. I just felt like a scared child who was babysitting this little baby.

In many ways, this is the expected content and cadence of a birth story in the United States. The harrowing and the traumatic are standard features

DOI: 10.4324/9781003499428-1

of contemporary childbirths. What is perhaps unexpected is how Marion described her second birth three years later, in 2018. In her words:

> I just kept thinking the whole time "This so great! I can't believe I get to do this this time! I can't believe I get to *be in this* this time!" and [I'm] not missing any of it, and not, like, you know, hearing about it later. I'm experiencing every second and it's so great!

VBAC (vaginal birth after cesarean) is not embraced by many practicing obstetricians in spite of the ample scientific evidence of comparable safety for both the birthing person and for the neonate. Barring certain risk factors, VBACs have fully been proven to be as safe as other vaginal births and promise significant benefits (California Maternal Quality Care Collaborative [CMQCC], 2022). Finding obstetricians who are willing to care for and to support a VBAC in a hospital can be difficult for many birthing people who are seeking to avoid repeat cesareans and their associated risks: only about half succeed in so doing (CMQCC, 2022). But Marion had not been deterred. This time she'd prepared for her second birth with consistent, high-quality, and personalized midwifery care. With this care, she successfully navigated the avoidable risks. For example, upon a thorough review of her medical records, her midwife found that Marion had tested positive for Group B Streptococcus (GBS) during her first pregnancy; no one had informed or counseled Marion about it. GBS is a common, harmless member of the gastrointestinal and genital microbiomes that can come and go. Unfortunately, GBS poses risks during pregnancy. For example, GBS increases the likelihood of perinatal complications including preterm prelabor rupture of membranes (PPROM) which is what had landed Marion in the hospital during her first birth. PPROM affects around 1% of pregnancies overall—although it is twice as likely for Black women in the US (Dayal & Hong, 2024). With her midwife's guidance, Marion was able to take measures to reduce these GBS risks and to improve her overall wellbeing throughout her pregnancy, including her diet, exercise, and other lifestyle factors. After a healthy, happy pregnancy, she gave birth physiologically, full term and without complications or interventions in an autonomous birth center with the support of her regular midwife, a doula, and her partner. Here is what she said about her experience:

> I would totally do it again, like right now! … When she (my baby) was born, I mean, that high is insane! ... Talk about pleasure. I've never done drugs, but—I'll do birth! ... if you could bottle that stuff!

Marion's joyful words may strike the reader as implausible, even outrageous, but her experience was echoed in varied tones during many of my interviews, for example:

> "I haven't felt anything so intense, so beautiful—ever." Nava
>
> "I remember feeling really good about it. ... it's kind of like being on ecstasy... Everything was beautiful. It was just light and airy, and like, a floating kind of feeling." Julia
>
> "I was surrounded by people who I trusted. It was just, like, *love overflow*. It sounds so cheesy, but it was just like that, such a warm feeling. And then it was August, and it was hot and sunny. It was just perfect." Melissa
>
> "I didn't feel any pain ... I felt joy. I really was happy. In my soul, in my cells, in my heart. I just felt so peaceful. It was a beautiful morning." Chandra
>
> "I could really see how it [pleasure] opened me. You know? And, and the mixture of that intensity, it was almost hard to tell the difference between the pleasure and pain." Venus
>
> "*That's not a thing!*" Male leader in women's sexual medicine

When I was just beginning this research, I attended the conference of a well-respected organization that is focused on women's sexual health. As a new member, I stood at the welcome table hoping that making some new connections might help me feel less awkward. Over walks the man who had just been speaking at the keynote podium: the current president. Looking at my belly, he begins.by asking me: "So, how far along?" After the prerequisite pregnancy-related pleasantries, he then asked: "So, what do you do?" I told him that I was a doctoral student beginning a study of pleasure in birth. "*That's not a thing!*" he snapped angrily at me. The others at the table stopped their chatting and looked over at us. I assured him that I was studying pleasure in birth in part because I had experienced it myself. "I've spent my career repairing the damage birth does to women," he said through gritted teeth. He looked me over then turned his attention to others without another word. I had clearly tripped a wire. Then and there I doubled down on my commitment to see this research through. The result is this book, a culmination of over eight years of study, analyses, and the lived experiences of myself and many others.

The wire that I had tripped had something to do with power, the compromised positioning of pregnant bodies, and the intersecting social forces acting upon and within these bodies—including mine. I was confronting forces I lacked words for but was discovering in real time. In her recent work on the policing and the criminalization of pregnant people, Grace Howard coined the term *pregnancy exceptionalism* to convey how “Pregnant people occupy a different, lower space in the United States’ system of law,” (and I would add in society in general) (2024, p. 3). This term captures what I couldn’t quite name then, how I found myself in a realm somehow separate from a standard form of full personhood or full citizenship. Surveillance, assessment, commentary, management, and control over my body by others (professionals or everyday strangers) were rendered expectable and enforceable. In this *exceptional* realm, I found, in ways big and small, that my rights, or perhaps my “right to have rights” as aptly put by Hannah Arendt (2024, p. 316), was fundamentally altered in some way by my physiological state. This alteration was particularly palpable inside biomedical institutions; on reading Arendt (dealing with what she called: “the calamity of statelessness”) I found myself struck in the gut:

> The fundamental deprivation of human rights is manifested first and above all in the deprivation of a *place* in the world which makes *opinions significant* and *actions effective*.
>
> *(Arendt, 2024, p. 315, emphasis mine)*

She then continued:

> Before this, what we must call a “human right,” today would have been thought of as a general characteristic of the human condition which no tyrant could take away. Its loss entails the loss of the *relevance of speech*...and the *loss of all human relationship*...the loss, in other words, of some of the most essential characteristics of human life.
>
> *(Arendt, 2024, p. 316, emphasis mine)*

Arendt’s words resonate with many of the experiences of the birthing people whom I have spoken with and have formally interviewed: birth plans ripped up and thrown in the trash right before their eyes, companionship by doulas, partners, or family being restricted or denied entirely, basic requests casually ignored, informed consent regularly overridden by manipulation or violence. Pregnancy and birth are states during which childbearers frequently take on a separate and an inferior status, wherein the places that they are often compelled to occupy render their *opinions insignificant and their actions ineffective*. Perhaps it is the status of “human being” that is rescinded while childbearers are pregnant, with both pregnancy and birth engendering an uncomfortable liminal space that has been well-articulated by Robbie Davis-Floyd (2022).

Arendt strongly insisted that: "...we really have begun to live in One World" (2024, p. 316). This "One World," or a realm that I'd myself been confronting, like so many others, is what Barbara Katz Rothman has called the: *Biomedical Empire*:

> Biomedicine is not only a profession, a discipline, a set of industries, or even a cluster of professions, disciplines and industries; biomedicine now functions *globally* much the way we have always understood imperial powers to function ... It is no longer medicine as a profession, but biomedicine as an industry that exerts power and controls its distribution. And it will always be done in a way that benefits the industry, the system, the Empire ... *Biomedical imperialism is one of the strongest forces on earth today.*"
>
> *(Katz Rothman, 2021, pp. 23–24, emphasis mine)*

My pregnancy had somehow altered my status as human, and thereby my *right to have rights* by my exclusion from the standard notion of a human being into a distinct class that is often subjected to governance in a particular style under biomedicine's authority. Experiencing pregnancy and *pregnancy exceptionalism* (Howard, 2024), *rightlessness* (Arendt, 2024) as a subject of the *Biomedical Empire* while in the midst of my doctoral program had a way of reorienting my scholarship. The more I studied and experienced pregnancy, birth culture, and perinatal care structures and institutions, the more this power hierarchy loomed over me and the more alienated I felt. Within myself, I was full of joy and brimming with new and unfolding kinds of power, but the external world was at odds with this joy. The deep, experiential knowledge of pregnancy by birthing people was absent everywhere I looked for it. Instead, that knowledge was merely about us, imposed on us, directed at us, done to us, but was not truly our own.

Perhaps nowhere is *pregnancy exceptionalism* as evident and the *Biomedical Empire* made so palpable as in childbirth. Childbirth is a trigger-point for many violations of birthing people's autonomy, consent, privacy, and basic human rights, particularly for historically and presently oppressed groups. The right to reproduce is fundamental to human dignity. In reality, this right functions rather as a privilege constrained along the lines of race, class, gender, sexuality, ability, and disability. Dorothy Roberts' *Killing the Black Body*, now well past its 20th anniversary (2017), remains vital to this analysis of power, tracing eugenic ideologies that continue to animate the policies and practices that control reproduction and strip Black and other marginalized birthing people of a powerful aspect of their human dignity. The "gates of life" as Katz Rothman has described them, hold unique potency within the human story:

> Birth and death aren't procedures, something for which the existentially constant you suits up, deals, and comes through the other end. They are definitionally transformative. You will never be the same. The one of you will be two. Or none. And the people who love you—they will never be the same. Your spouse will be a parent or will be widowed. Your parent will be a grandparent or bereaved beyond measure. Your child will be a sibling or an orphan.
>
> *(Katz Rothman, 2021, p. 80)*

My pregnancy and birth repositioned my solidarity, my allegiances, everything about me expanding, contracting, churning, rebelling. I felt how, at all points in the reproductive life course, biomedical power was to be appeased as the ultimate grantor of truth and legitimacy. The "Biomedical Empire" had (and continues to) arbitrate life itself, death itself, personhood, and ultimately reality—a reality that has frowned upon and that has stolen the joy from birth. I launched into my research with the goal of giving primacy to birthing people's experiences in their fullness as opposed to, for example, the views of their care providers and the institutions and systems that they occupy. I realize now that I'd sought to defy misery, if only in my own curiosity. This defiance felt really good.

The study of pleasure is effortlessly and delightfully controversial, and this is particularly true of the pleasure of women and femmes, queer people, and those with the capacity for pregnancy as a whole. Feeling good is naughty, isn't it? Pleasure, which is a massive category of sensations and experiences, is typically pigeon-holed into sexual definitions, which saddles this very important topic with all of the baggage of the repressive sexual cultural mores that are still dominant in the United States and elsewhere. Focusing on pleasure also defies both the implicit and explicit rules that have been placed on the seriousness of scholarly inquiry. Certainly, pain is more important. Is it not frivolous and insulting to focus on pleasure when there is so much suffering? In short, no. It is precisely the pressure not to focus on pleasure that had hinted to me that there were untapped radical potentials along this line of inquiry. To be frank, my own experience of pleasure in the crucible of childbirth was an indelible and transformative moment in my life. Birth provoked in me a profound curiosity and gave me a distinct lens to explore and analyze birth culture. When I have mentioned my work to other birthing people it has prompted intrigue and gratitude. While most people I've spoken to have had no idea that pleasure was a possibility in childbirth, many told me they'd secretly had birth experiences like mine but told next to no one about them. That drew me in further. Also, and importantly, my self-care during my postpartum period required my careful choice regarding what I would study. I unapologetically chose pleasure for myself.

Pleasure, Praxis, and Birth Research

The few published studies on birth pleasure have focused on "obstetrical orgasm" as the preeminent iteration of pleasure during the birthing process, the value of which is based primarily upon the potential for pain relief (Mayberry & Daniel, 2016; Postel, 2013). Pleasure on its own merit hasn't been addressed. Buckley and Dip (2003) and Khajehei and Doherty (2012) came to similar conclusions during their literature reviews. They described the hormonal aspects of birth physiology and the negative impacts of the various intrapartum biomedical interventions into the birthing process on the birthing person's levels of oxytocin, beta-endorphins, catecholamines, and prolactin, which are related to both sexual pleasure and to the birth process.

The disparities between birth experiences and birth-related health outcomes have been well-documented across racial and class markers, with high rates of maternal morbidities and mortalities among racialized and economically marginalized women, and with Black women presently facing roughly a four-fold risk of maternal mortality as compared to White women (Centers for Disease Control and Prevention [CDC], 2023; Crear-Perry et al., 2021; Lu et al., 2010; MacDorman et al., 2016; Oparah et al., 2016, Oparah and Bonaparte, 2015; World Health Organization [WHO], 2021). The few studies of birth pleasure thus far have engaged almost exclusively with affluent White participants. In their powerful, engaged intersectional anti-racist Black feminist analysis of Black childbearers' experiences of birth (albeit not birth pleasure), Julia Chinyere Oparah and the Black Women Birthing Justice (BWBJ) collective had carefully catalogued the many ways in which Black women are currently being forced to battle for their bodily autonomy and for choices in birth because of intersecting racism and sexism (2016). The birth experiences of People of Color are absent from the past academic work on birth pleasure, a gap that my study addresses head on.

Despite the dearth of peer-reviewed academic work on this important topic, some researchers have acknowledged and have promoted pleasure as an important aspect of birth. The Midwifery Model of Care (MMOC)

(Katz Rothman, 1982) has long emphasized both pleasure and sensuality during birth (for a full description of the MMOC, see Davis-Floyd, 2018). Midwifery texts on pre- and intrapartum care have extensively addressed both birth pleasures and sexuality (for example, see Walsh & Downe, 2013). Ina May Gaskin, who is possibly the most influential midwife in the world today, has informed generations of lay readers about the existence of birth pleasure in her three still widely read books: Spiritual Midwifery (2010), Ina May's Guide to Childbirth (2008), and Birth Matters: A Midwife's Manifesta (2011). Over a decade ago, the also world-famous doula and doula trainer Debra Pascali Bonaro's 2008 documentary film: *Orgasmic Birth: The Best-Kept Secret* was released to the public. The fascinating and very informative film was followed by the book *Orgasmic Birth: Your Guide to a Safe, Satisfying, and Pleasurable Birth Experience* (Davis & Pascali Bonaro, 2010), which has become popular in "natural childbirth" preparation circles. Just a handful of peer-reviewed studies have addressed the existence of birth pleasure, which have framed this phenomenon predominantly as "obstetric orgasm" (Buckley, 2010; Caffrey, 2014; Mayberry & Daniel, 2016; Postel, 2013). The orgasmic birth model tends to be interpreted as emphasizing sexual pleasure. Other nonsexual or nonorgasmic iterations of birth pleasure are not emphasized. Given the gaps in the research around pleasure in the birthing process, I studied birth pleasure in its heterogeneity, and its relationships to birthing people's overall wellbeing.

Birthing people and society at large shape and are shaped by births, in a form of micro- and macro-level praxis (Cheyney, 2008) and worldmaking (Goodman, 1978). "Praxis" can be understood as the reciprocal and mutually reinforcing process of reflection and action, taking ideas and analyses to transform these into practical applications, utilizing these practical experiences to generate analyses and theories for change-making and liberation (Cho et al., 2013; Freire, 1970). "Worldmaking" refers to the process of conjuring relative, context-dependent realities, real or imaginary (see Nelson Goodman's 1978 work, *Ways of Worldmaking*). Social forces are apparent in and greatly impact the birth experience itself as well as birth outcomes, which track social hierarchical gradients such as race and class (Blumenshine et al., 2010; Crear-Perry et al., 2021). Countless biomedical, public health, sociological, and anthropological studies of birth have been published over the decades. None have directly dealt with birth pleasure as a sociocultural phenomenon with relationships to race, class, or gender. This study is among the first to examine birth pleasure within the context of social power and in relationship to birth justice. Next, I want to highlight the fundamental scholarship on birth culture that has deeply informed my research.

Brigitte Jordan's (1993) landmark anthropological book *Birth in Four Cultures* (the United States, the Yucatán Maya, Sweden, and Holland) highlighted the ways in which cultures produce birthing systems that comport with and propagate their values, beliefs, and hegemonic power structures (see Davis-Floyd, 2022, for multiple examples of these phenomena). Although Jordan hadn't specifically addressed pleasure in birth she (1993) advanced a "biosocial" model of birth that engages the body and culture as one, which has been a foundational concept for my study (p. 48). Jordan's work was expanded upon in Robbie Davis-Floyd's and Melissa Cheyney's 2019 publication *Birth in Eight Cultures*. The ethnographies that these coeditors had included therein were engaged in cross-comparative analyses to make visible the often-invisible forces of culture in birth-giving spaces. Pleasure, however, was seldom mentioned in this book. One of the eight chapters that these two coeditors had chosen to include in their book had focused on the ethnographic analysis of the United States's birth culture as contrasted against that of the Netherlands (Cheyney et al., 2019), and centered on the value systems, beliefs, structures, and practices of differing kinds of care providers, including professional midwives and biomedical obstetricians and gynecologists. These coauthors concluded that even while the biomedical model of birth enjoys near total control in the United States "community midwives and the families who seek their care today are still struggling to carve out a small niche within this deeply entrenched technocratic US hospital birth monopoly" (Cheyney et al., 2019, p. 184). These coauthors called for changes in birth care paradigms that would make "childbirth emotionally meaningful and medically safe for all" (Cheyney et al., 2019, p. 200). I want to note here that the ever-present appeals to "biomedical safety" within the birth research serve to reinforce the dominance of the *Biomedical Empire* in a bid for both practical and narrative validity (Katz Rothman, 2021).

Davis-Floyd's (2022) third edition of *Birth as an American Rite of Passage* was based on a comparative study of American births from the viewpoints of 65 birthing women who'd given birth at any time after the year 2000, and of 100 women who'd given birth during the late 1990s. Davis-Floyd described the "technocratic," "humanistic," and "holistic" models/paradigms of birth and health care, and the extreme differences among these three paradigms. She also detailed the standard biomedicalized birth routines, which she'd interestingly analyzed as actually being "rituals" that enact, display, and transmit the core values and beliefs of multiple technocratic societies. Davis-Floyd additionally described the usually unnecessary rituals/biomedical interventions into the birthing process that had been and are still being all too frequently performed under the influence of the still-hegemonic technocratic model. Davis-Floyd also provided strong evidence that these standardized routines/rituals are resistant to change (despite the ample scientific evidence of their harmfulness, and the near-total absence of scientific evidence proving their safety) because this again still-hegemonic model serves cultural functions that had been and continue to be of great importance to patriarchal, biomedical, and technological powers. Her argument is that birth-related medical interventions can be better understood as *rituals*, and technocratic birth specifically can be understood as a *rite of passage* that serves the interests of the American patriarchy and of the US biomedical establishment more than it does those of birthing people and their newborns. Davis-Floyd had additionally argued that these rituals serve to contain the many threatening elements of the birth process that contradict American cultural values and beliefs (such as individualism, man and technology over nature, man over woman, mind over body, more over less) and transform the pregnant not-yet-mother into "American motherhood," which is a social construct born of and in service to the US patriarchy, capitalism, militarism, and nationalism. Davis-Floyd (2022) argued that technocratic birth trains new mothers to surrender themselves and their children to the powerful institutions that surround them—first, the biomedical institutions, then educational, and eventually the capitalist, industrial, and militaristic. Regarding sexual pleasure in birth, Davis-Floyd concluded that "so effective are hospital routines at masking the intense sexuality of birth that most women today are not even aware of birth's sexual nature" (p. 96). The "de-sexualization of birth" (pp. 33, 96) is so complete under the ongoing hegemony of this technocratic model (and the model itself is entirely hegemonic in framing birth as a biomedical accomplishment rather than as a formative human experience) that birth is not commonly recognized as part of the sexual life course let alone as a complex process with a myriad of physical and emotional facets, including pleasure. The slash in "OB/GYN" is functional as well as metaphorical: it conceptually divides off the sexual life and body from the pregnant and birthing body. I lean on Davis-Floyd's corpus of work with much gratitude throughout this book.

I leverage Katz Rothman's useful analyses as well. Her work on homebirth activism and scholarship has articulated the history, contours, and fissures of biomedicine, nurse-midwifery, community midwifery, and birth culture in the United States. A homebirth mother herself, Katz Rothmans' work leverages her positionality both as birthing-person and as a very well-known and highly respected sociologist. In *A Bun in the Oven*, she contrasted the food justice movement and the natural birth movement in how they both challenge the norms of hegemonic industrialization that invade the most intimate crevices of our lives. I have already drawn on her more recent work *The Biomedical Empire: Lessons Learned from the*

COVID-19 Pandemic, wherein Katz Rothman offered a useful analysis of how the COVID-19 pandemic has laid bare the imperialism of both the biomedical and the public health industries, operating as its own global empire within and beyond the nation-state. This Empire, she also argued, engages in pervasive colonization. External and internalized behavioral control of its citizens is based on a near religiosity of beliefs, with capitalist profit-making as its core motive. She also argued that human life and personhood itself have come to be defined, disciplined, and controlled by this Biomedical Empire, from the conception and the definition of a person to death, signing off on the literal bookends of our existence, from birth certificates to death certificates. *The Biomedical Empire* provides a useful heuristic for how power operates through birth in the United States, which I've put to work during my intersectional analyses.

Intersectionality

Intersectionality is a knowledge project that was first developed by Kimberely Crenshaw (1989) and that considers race, class, sexual orientation, gender, and other socially constructed systems and ideologies of hierarchy and power that do not exist or exert influence in isolation, but rather intersect, interact, and construct each other (Collins, 2015; Crenshaw, 1989). Although the United States spends more money than does any other high-income country (HIC) on obstetric care, nevertheless, in this HIC, maternal mortality has steadily increased since 2000, while over this same period of time, it has also steadily declined around the world (CDC, 2023; Hoyert, 2022; MacDorman et al., 2016; WHO, 2015). As I've previously mentioned, the US maternal mortality rate most intensely impacts Women of Color and impoverished women (Oparah et al., 2016). These facts are unintelligible without an intersectional lens that addresses race, class, gender, and the myriad of other social forces that are currently at play within maternal health. Therefore, it is important to re-examine how researchers study birthing people and childbirth. First, we must look directly to birthing people and their experiences. Second, by fully incorporating the embodied knowledge and the social realities of birthing people into our social science research works, we can fundamentally reimagine maternal health research and care. I also firmly believe that by following the lead of Black and Brown women and gender expansive birthing people is how this maternal health care crisis will be solved.

I will continue to cite and to highlight the multiple works of critical race reproductive justice scholars including Dorothy Roberts, Loretta Ross, Julia Chinyere Oparah, Black Women Birthing Justice (BWBJ), SisterSong (2022), and others. The status of Black women as mothers is more often questioned and targeted both legally and socially that is that of White women. Due to the pervasive and ongoing institutional and structural racism within health care, social services, and policing, Black women more than any other group are far too often declared as being "unfit" and as being a "danger to their child," and are also far too frequently reported to Social Services or to the US criminal justice system (Howard, 2024; Roberts, 2017). When Black women refuse a particular biomedical intervention in birth, they are much more likely than are White women to be labeled as "uncooperative" or as "combative" patients—labels that can be and often are used to trigger institutional assertions of power over their bodies, such as compelled mental health evaluations or drug testing (Flavin, 2008; Paltrow & Flavin, 2013; Roberts, 2017).

"Mother Blame" narratives that circulate around healthcare settings are a functional outgrowth of obstetric racism that I also firmly insist must be transformed (Davis, 2019; Scott et al., 2019). Doulas who support both White and Black clients have a powerful vantage point from which to observe, speak on, and resist systemic and obstetric racism in maternal health care, particularly Black doulas navigating biomedicalized birth spaces (Salinas et al., 2022). I additionally strongly insist that their knowledge and experiences must be incorporated into efforts for change. Some advocates have experimented with community-grounded models of birth support volunteers based in a birth justice framework (Kivlighan et al., 2022). Scott (2021) credited such movements for birth justice by Black women with an upswell of Black feminist intellectualism that she argued is essential for eliminating racism from maternal care and for improving health outcomes for Black mothers and birthing people. I also firmly suggest that models of birth care, from hospital-based to homebirth midwifery, must be interrogated for their systemic oppressions and should most definitely be transformed through a diversity of practical and effective tactics.

Although pleasure has seldom been investigated in maternal health, reproductive justice activists are presently and bravely leaning into conversations about joy and pleasure as forms of strong resistance to this current and ongoing biomedical hegemony (Francis, 2021). Given what is known about birth, the impacts of social support and stressors, fear, abuse, and the lack of control and autonomy that are also currently being experienced by many birthing people (of course, hierarchically graded upon these intersecting racial and class statuses and relative privileges), it is not a huge leap to postulate that oppressive systems of social forces show up during the birth process in ways that greatly inhibit birthing people's abilities to experience various types of pleasure during their births. Beyond, around, and imbuing all of that is the all-reaching "Biomedical Empire" and its ongoing dominance over the "gates of life," and indeed of personhood itself. In this book, I highlight multiple opportunities for improving maternity care and both birth and health outcomes, particularly for those who are most at risk under the current biomedical and still-hegemonic paradigm—Black, Brown, Indigenous, economically disenfranchised, gender-expansive mothers and parents, and other historically oppressed groups. Pleasure in birth and anywhere else, may just be what reproductive justice feels like. When suffering is the norm, feeling good is a rebellion.

This book is an invitation to its readers to deeply think about the disruptive potential of feeling good. The following pages present and contextualize my doctoral work examining the birth experiences of my study's participants, and the transgressive implications of experiencing pleasure during birth, both within and outside of healthcare institutions. The mixed-methods anthropological study that I present herein dove into what makes or breaks pleasurable birth experiences. My ethnographic interviews with 23 interlocutors, mostly People of Color of varied backgrounds and genders, covered 43 distinct birth experiences, many pleasurable, some not. My exploratory, non-probabilistic online survey of 1,781 participants (which I'd designed based on my interview data and had collaboratively refined with these interlocutors) gathered 578 written accounts and is the first quantitative study of pleasure during birth. For the sake of scope and length, this book centers the in-depth qualitative findings that I'd engaged through my sociocultural and intersectional analyses. For more on the particulars, refer to Appendix A, which is where I've described my study methodologies in detail.

To allow for a critical engagement with the study findings that follow, I first provide a crisp review and analysis of the historical roots of the birth culture in the United States. Then, I analyze these interlocutors' experiences of birth pleasure holistically and collectively through an intersectional lens. Next, I shift gears to chapters that hone in on specific power differentials across identities such as sexuality, gender, race, and class, as they weave together. My goal is to attend with care to the many facets of these differences, while avoiding as best I possibly can essentializations and/or over-generalizations, while at the same time tracing the threads of shared experience that weave throughout these data in ways that I hope may be useful to birthing people and to those who care for them.

Chapter Summaries

Chapter 1. Why We Give Birth This Way

This chapter covers the historical grounding that is necessary for a meaningful cultural analysis of birth in the United States—a necessary precondition for interpreting the findings of this study going forward. This historical sketch has included the ways in which the biomedicalization of birth unfolded, the cultural and political intersections with social justice movements along the way, and the long-reaching ramifications of those histories. This brief but thorough history of birth culture in the United States will allow my readers to better understand the invisible narratives that undergird the hegemonic approaches to childbirth care, to analyze the social and cultural forces that are currently at play, and to reckon with the costs of maintaining these established birth care structures, thereby making the case for the transformation of birth care on every level.

Chapter 2. Birth Pleasure Experiences and Perceptions

Herein, I present the main findings of my qualitative work in *The Birth Pleasure Study*, which revealed that both pleasure and pain are multidimensional and integral aspects of birth experiences, can co-arise, and are not mutually exclusive. This chapter covers the kinds of pleasures that can be experienced during childbirth by type, including emotional, mental, spiritual, physical, and sexual pleasures, and how these experiences of pleasures had been perceived by these study participants. To help my readers to understand these varied expressions of pleasures, I developed a "Typology of Birth Pleasure," which will help to frame my readers' thinking going forward into the rest of this text.

Chapter 3. Pain-Free Birth

"Pain-free birth" might sound like an oxymoron. In this study, roughly half of my interview participants reported experiences of birth that'd been pain-free in whole or in part (and typically without any pain-alleviating medications). This chapter goes into depth about these experiences, how they were fostered, and what they meant to those who experienced them. Some of these pain-free births had occurred unexpectedly, but often these experiences had been the result of intentional and even intensive preparation and training, such as in the cases of those who'd carefully practiced hypnobirthing or meditative techniques. For some of these study participants, aspects of birth they were expecting to be painful simply hadn't been. Finally, I analyze the pain-free experience of one participant's induction without an epidural or analgesia for almost her entire labor, but then had an epidural placed in preparation for an emergency cesarean birth (CB) before having discovered that she was already fully dilated. The intention of this chapter is not to establish some new ideal birth to which birthing people must aspire. Rather, my goal is to document and to fully articulate these pain-free birth experiences as valid, and as having been somewhat akin to documenting the impossible, both to challenge and to expand what is hegemonically known and believed about birth.

Chapter 4. Medicalization, De-medicalization, and Praxis

This chapter covers pleasurable birth experiences within medicalized and de-medicalized contexts and explores praxis across a spectrum of medicalization in childbirth. Herein, I frame medicalization as a mindset, rather than a characteristic of any particular birth. Rather than assigning "medicalized" or "de-medicalized" categorizations to the study participants' experiences (based on my own assessment of their birth setting, interventions, or the procedures that had been employed), I instead have privileged the participant's view of their own birth. I start with those who viewed their births as fundamentally medical events and then move to those who shifted their views (which had gone only in the direction of de-medicalization), and finally to those who rebuked a biomedical frame for all of their birth experiences. To conclude, I present additional analyses of those who'd not only had a de-medicalized mindset toward their births but had fully relished in them, thereby deriving a particular kind of birth pleasure, pleasure in defiance, as a praxis for strongly challenging the biomedical power over their birthing bodies.

Chapter 5. The Sexuality Connection in Birth

In this chapter, I address the relationships between sexuality and pleasurable birth experiences, illustrating both how sexuality impacted birth, and how birth impacted sexuality. I focus on how the interview participants related their pleasurable birthing experiences to their personal sexual relationships and their sexual lives by incorporating how concepts of gender, sexism, and sexual identity had emerged during these interviews. Some interlocutors dealt with both sexist and cisheteronormative oppressions. I found that a birthing person's sexual orientation had also involved a range of both oppressive and liberating energies during their birth, particularly for those who'd given birth in their own home and thus had more latitude for relational or even sexual expressions. I analyze the role that sex played during labor and birth, focusing on those participants who'd had sex during their early labor or just before their labor had started. Lastly, I tackle the three remaining themes regarding sexuality during the aftermath of pleasurable birth: personal sexual empowerment, physiologic changes, and relational factors.

Chapter 6. Race, Class, and Feeling Good in Birth

This chapter covers the ways race and class intersected in birthing people's experiences of birth pleasure, specifically how the interview participants connected their experiences of pleasure during birth to their racial identities and class positionalities. Herein, I group the participants by how they defined themselves in terms of race. Calling on the subversive tenor of Nina Simone's iconic song "Feeling Good," I do my best to convey the rebellion that was woven into the embodiment of pleasure for birth-giving people, especially those of historically marginalized racialized and classed identities. By grouping participants by race, I aim not to flatten down complexities but rather to interrogate deeper nuances. I also explore the differences in how racism and classism have impacted my study participants and address the patterns that had emerged within racial categories as well as far beyond them.

Chapter 7. The Pleasure-Forward Birth Model

In this chapter I present The Pleasure-Forward Birth Model, a preliminary framework for implementing and building on the findings of my research in the movement toward reproductive justice. At the center is the birthing person's experience. I also describe the relational, contextual, and structural layers that surround and permeate the birth space, thereby impacting the birthing person. I propose that birth pleasure may be a symptom of birth going well, a salutogenic signal that reinforces birth physiology. This model contrasts with the "biomedical cascade of interventions," the problematic and routine overuse of biomedical interventions in birth which in a vicious cycle build on each other and move toward increased odds of cesarean birth that might have otherwise been avoidable (Davis-Floyd 2022, pp. 13–14; Tracy et al., 2007). Herein, I propose that a cascade of positive, pleasurable experiences can build toward heightened birth wellbeing in a virtuous cycle. Support for and barriers to birth pleasure are predictably patterned by sociocultural powers. This chapter concludes the book with some syntheses, a discussion of my study's limitations, and this study's implications for birthing people and for those who are fighting for reproductive justice, thereby rendering the praxis of birth-giving as worldmaking.

References

Arendt, H. (2024). *The origins of totalitarianism.* Mariner Classics. (Original 1949, Harcourt Brace).

Buckley, S. J., & Dip, O. (2003, Summer). Undisturbed birth: Nature's blueprint for ease and ecstasy. *Journal of Prenatal and Perinatal Psychology and Health, 17*, 261–288. www.birthpsychology.com/wp-content/uploads/journal/published_paper/volume-17/issue-4/06xgsNya.pdf

Buckley, S. J. (2010). Sexuality in labour and birth: An intimate perspective. In D. Walsh & S. Downe (Eds.), *Essential midwifery practice: Intrapartum care* (pp. 213–234). Blackwell. https://doi.org/10.1002/9781444317701.ch12

Blumenshine, P., Egerter, S., Barclay, C. J., Cubbin, C., & Braveman, P. A. (2010). Socioeconomic disparities in adverse birth outcomes: A systematic review. *American Journal of Preventive Medicine*, *39*(3), 263–272. https://doi.org/10.1016/j.amepre.2010.05.012

Caffrey, A. (2014). Experiences of pleasurable childbirth: Uncovering a blind spot in anthropology. *Popular Anthropology Magazine*, *5*(1), 17–27. www.popanthro.org/index.php/PopAnthro/article/download/145/147

CDC & National Center for Health Statistics (2023). *Births–Method of Delivery*. FastStats Homepage. www.cdc.gov/nchs/fastats/delivery.htm

Cheyney, M. J. (2008). Homebirth as systems-challenging praxis: Knowledge, power, and intimacy in the birthplace. *Qualitative Health Research*, *18*(2), 254–267. https://doi.org/10.1177/1049732307312393

Cheyney, M. J., Goodarzi, B., Wiegers, T., Davis-Floyd, R., & Vedam, S. (2019). Giving birth in the United States and The Netherlands: Midwifery care as integrated option or contested privilege? In R. Davis-Floyd & M. J. Cheyney (Eds.), *Birth in eight cultures* (pp. 165–202). Waveband Press.

Cho, S., Crenshaw, K. W., & McCall, L. (2013). Toward a field of intersectionality studies: Theory, applications, and praxis. *Signs: Journal of Women in Culture and Society*, *38*(4), 785–810. https://doi.org/10.1086/669608

California Maternal Quality Care Collaborative (2022, November 30). *Toolkit to Support Vaginal Birth and Reduce Primary Cesareans, Addended 2022*. www.cmqcc.org/content/toolkit-support-vaginal-birth-and-reduce-primary-cesareans-addended-2022

Collins, P. H. (2015). Intersectionality's definitional dilemmas. *Annual Review of Sociology*, *41*, 1–20. https://doi.org/10.1146/annurev-soc-073014-112142

Crear-Perry, J., Correa-de-Araujo, R., Lewis Johnson, T., McLemore, M. R., Neilson, E., & Wallace, M. (2021). Social and structural determinants of health inequities in maternal health. *Journal of Women's Health*, *30*(2), 230–235. https://doi.org/10.1089/jwh.2020.8882

Crenshaw, K. (1989). Demarginalizing the intersection of race and sex: A Black feminist critique of antidiscrimination doctrine, feminist theory and antiracist politics. *University of Chicago Legal Forum*, *1989*(1), 139–167. http://chicagounbound.uchicago.edu/uclf/vol1989/iss1/8

Davis, D. A. (2019). Obstetric racism: The racial politics of pregnancy, labor, and birthing. *Medical Anthropology*, *38*(7), 560–573. https://doi.org/10.1080/01459740.2018.1549389

Davis, E., & Pascali Bonaro, D. (2010). Orgasmic birth: Your guide to a safe, satisfying, and pleasurable birth experience. Rodale.

Davis-Floyd, R. (2018). *Ways of knowing about birth: Mothers, midwives, medicine, and birth activism*. Waveland Press.

Davis-Floyd, R. (2022). *Birth as an American rite of passage* (3rd ed.). Routledge.

Davis-Floyd, R., & Cheyney, M. (Eds.). (2019). *Birth in eight cultures*. Waveland Press.

Dayal, S., Jenkins, S. M., & Hong, P. L. (2024). Preterm and term prelabor rupture of membranes (PPROM and PROM). In *StatPearls*. StatPearls Publishing.

Flavin, J. (2008). *Our bodies, our crimes: The policing of women's reproduction in America*. NYU Press.

Francis, C. E. (2021). *A real hot girl movement: A social history of pleasure activism in Atlanta, Georgia* [Doctoral dissertation, California Institute of Integral Studies]. ProQuest Dissertations and Theses Global.

Freire, P. (1970). *Pedagogy of the oppressed*. (M. Bergman Ramos, Trans.). Continuum.

Gaskin, I. M. (2008). *Ina May's guide to childbirth: Updated with new material*. Bantam.

Gaskin, I. M. (2010). *Spiritual midwifery*. Book Publishing Company.

Gaskin, I. M. (2011). *Birth matters: A midwife's manifesta*. Seven Stories Press.

Goodman, N. (1978). *Ways of worldmaking*. Hackett.

Howard, G. (2024). *The pregnancy police: Conceiving crime, arresting personhood*. University of California Press.

Hoyert, D. L. (2022). Maternal mortality rates in the United States, 2020. *NCHS Health E-Stats*. https://doi.org/10.15620/cdc:113967

Jordan, B. (1993). *Birth in four cultures: A crosscultural investigation of childbirth in Yucatan, Holland, Sweden, and the United States* (4th ed.). Waveland Press.

Katz Rothman, B. (1982). *In labor: Women and power in the birthplace* (1st ed.). Norton.

Katz Rothman, B. (2021). *The biomedical empire: Lessons learned from the COVID-19 pandemic*. Stanford University Press.

Khajehei, M., & Doherty, M. (2012). Childbirth in pleasure and ecstasy: A fountain of hormones and chemicals. *International Journal of Childbirth Education*, *27*(3). https://search.ebscohost.com/login.aspx?direct=true&profile=ehost&scope=site&authtype=crawler&jrnl=08878625&AN=82251209&h=s1G1O0r%2Ftq10UcTYXwGvZ4FK1iU2wu7l%2BlOtfTDyaDCtnEozhzDLR1dqwR2KoAIBRFslShyL9OoC84dceP0gzw%3D%3D&crl=c

Kivlighan, K. T., Gardner, T., Murphy, C., Reiss, P., Griffin, C., & Migliaccio, L. (2022). Grounded in community: Development of a birth justice-focused volunteer birth companion program. *Journal of Midwifery & Women's Health*, *67*, 740–745. https://doi.org/10.1111/jmwh.13407

Lu, M. C., Kotelchuck, M., Hogan, V., Jones, L., Wright, K., & Halfon, N. (2010). Closing the Black–White gap in birth outcomes: A life-course approach. *Ethnicity & Disease*, *20*(1 Suppl 2), S2–62–76. PMID: 20629248. www.ncbi.nlm.nih.gov/pmc/articles/PMC4443479/

MacDorman, M. F., Declercq, E., Cabral, H., & Morton, C. (2016). Is the United States maternal mortality rate increasing? Disentangling trends from measurement issues. *Obstetrics and Gynecology*, *128*(3), 447–455. http://doi.org/10.1097/AOG.0000000000001556

Mayberry, L., & Daniel, J. (2016). "Birthgasm" A literary review of orgasm as an alternative mode of pain relief in childbirth. *Journal of Holistic Nursing*, *34*(4), 331–342. https://doi.org/10.1177/0898010115614205

Oparah, J. C., Arega, H., Hudson, D., Jones, L., & Oseguera, T. (2016). *Battling over birth: Black women and the maternal health care crisis in California*. Black Women Birthing Justice Report.

Oparah, J. C., & Black Women Birthing Justice. (2016). Beyond coersion and malign neglect: Black women and the struggle for birth justice, Introduction. In J. C. Oparah & A. D. Bonaparte (Eds.), *Birthing justice: Black women, pregnancy, and childbirth*. Routledge.

Oparah, J. C., & Bonaparte, A. D. (Eds.). (2015). *Birthing justice: Black women, pregnancy, and childbirth*. Routledge.

Paltrow, L. M., & Flavin, J. (2013). Arrests of and forced interventions on pregnant women in the United States, 1973–2005: Implications for women's legal status and public health. *Journal of Health Politics, Policy and Law*, 38(2), 299–343. https://doi.org/10.1215/03616878-1966324

Pascali Bonaro, D. (Director). (2008). *Orgasmic birth: The best-kept secret* [Film]. Sunken Treasure.

Postel, T. (2013). Childbirth climax: The revealing of obstetrical orgasm. *Sexologies*, *22*(4), e89–e92. https://doi.org/10.1016/j.sexol.2013.03.011

Roberts, D. (2017). *Killing the Black body: Race, reproduction, and the meaning of liberty* (2nd ed.). Vintage.

Salinas, J. L., Salinas, M., & Kahn, M. (2022). Doulas, racism, and Whiteness: How birth support workers process advocacy towards women of color. *Societies*, *12*(1), 19. https://doi.org/10.3390/soc12010019

Scott, K. A. (2021). The rise of Black feminist intellectual thought and political activism in perinatal quality improvement: A righteous rage about racism, resistance, resilience, and rigor. *Feminist Anthropology*, *2*(1), 155–160. https://doi.org/10.1002/fea2.12045

Scott, K. A., Britton, L., & McLemore, M. R. (2019). The ethics of perinatal care for black women: Dismantling the structural racism in "mother blame" narratives. *Journal of Perinatal & Neonatal Nursing*, *33*(2), 108–115. https://doi.org/10.1097/jpn.0000000000000394

SisterSong. (2022). *Reproductive justice*. www.sistersong.net/reproductive-justice

Tracy, S. K., Sullivan, E., Wang, Y. A., Black, D., & Tracy, M. (2007). Birth outcomes associated with interventions in labour amongst low risk women: A population-based study. Women and Birth, 20(2), 41–48. https://doi.org/10.1016/j.wombi.2007.03.005

Walsh, D., & Downe, S. (Eds.). (2013). *Intrapartum care*. John Wiley.

World Health Organization. (2015). UNICEF, UNFPA, World Bank Group, & United Nations Population Division. *Trends in maternal mortality: 1990–2015: REPORT.* www.unfpa.org/sites/default/files/pub-pdf/9789241565141_eng.pdf

World Health Organization. (2021). *WHO statement on caesarean section rates*. www.who.int/news-room/questions-and-answers/item/who-statement-on-caesarean-section-rates-frequently-asked-questions

1

WHY WE GIVE BIRTH THIS WAY

The maternal health crisis in the United States continues with largely worsening maternal health outcomes, increasing biomedical interventions into birthing processes, glaring and devastating racial disparities, vanishing care infrastructures, and study after study grappling with why. While the predominant mode of thinking and problem-solving of maternal health issues is biomedical, the reality of this crisis is grounded in the cultural and social layers that are often discussed in the literature in terms of demographics or competency rather than in terms of transformative praxis. I find myself working on "how" questions as I reflect on my own and the many pleasurable birth experiences that were so generously and courageously shared with me in my research. I am asked the same two questions when I share about my work with others: "Pleasure in birth? How?" I, too, want to know how. How can we make birth better? How do we do better? But these "how" questions walk hand in hand with "whys." Why do we birth in this way? Why is birth so traumatic, painful, and scary by default? Why is there so much interest in making birth tolerable, but such a strong aversion to the idea of birth being incredible? To engage these questions in the coming text, I now turn my attention to understand birth as a social construction and the historical roots of the hegemonic birth culture in the United States.

Birth as a Social Construction

Pain and fear are the dominant features in the social construction of birth within the current US context, which conceptualizes birth as a dangerous

DOI: 10.4324/9781003499428-2

medical event to be controlled by technologically advanced biomedicine (for multiple examples of this conceptualization, see Davis-Floyd & Premkumar, 2023a, 2023b, 2023c). Biomedicine generates and enforces these norms. In the US, popular discourses generally perpetuate birthing people's fears, their usual expectations of unfathomable pain, and their ignorance of other experiential possibilities during their births, particularly in the media (Leachman, 2017). These norms can be traced back to Judeo-Christian ideologies in the matter of childbirth, with pain the curse and punishment born by all women/birthing people for Eve's unforgivable pursuit of knowledge (Delaport, 2018; Thompson, 2019).

Socially constructed norms make their way into the embodied experiences of individuals via the psychosocial mechanisms of social cognitions and attitudes (Hogg et al., 2010). It follows that many birthing people relate to their births as being fearful, a dangerous "point of no return," that is often characterized by uncertainty, pain, and peril (Sheen & Spade, 2018; Wigert et al., 2020). Some childbearers have described even pathological levels of fear of birth, or tokophobia (Hofberg & Brockington, 2000). In one study of 8,000 women, 40% of respondents reported that they had feared pain during childbirth at a clinically significant level (Geissbuehler & Eberhard, 2002, p. 231), which fully corresponds with the hegemonic biomedical approaches to birth management (Davis-Floyd, 2003, 2022). During birth and beyond this context, pain conveys danger or harm, has profound psychological impacts, and can trigger past or present traumatic experiences (Creedy et al., 2000) in ways that all too often disrupt birth physiology.

Alternative constructions are effectively stifled when it comes to birth. Already, childbirth is a difficult or taboo topic for many. Rare conversations about birth often resemble the exchange of war stories among veterans. Without a social script to enable their articulations with others, positive birth stories are often withheld. Many of my interview participants said that they had never discussed their pleasurable birth experiences with anyone else before our interviews for fear of offending others or out of a sense of shame. Some interview participants shared that discussing their pleasurable birth experiences with me had been both transformative and healing for them. This silencing reinforces a birth culture that is currently centered on both pain and pathology over any other real experiential possibilities, such as pleasure, during birth.

And yet, and rather obviously, birth has existed long before colonization, capitalism, and global biomedical empire (Katz Rothman, 2021). Birth is many things to people: a cultural event, a spiritual event, a private family moment, a rite of passage, an adventure, or even an intimate romantic or erotic experience. Some people give birth completely free of pain—without analgesia. Some enjoy the sensations and experiences of birth. Others reject a pleasure-pain dichotomy and instead create entirely different frames of reference for their multiple birth sensations. It would seem countercultural to fully humanize (rather than dehumanize) birthing people by embracing their identities, unique pregnancies, histories, constellations of relationships, all of which are situated within their respective sociocultural contexts. Within the generally biomedical and industrialized birth culture within the United States context, humanization is often at odds with institutional operations. The flattening, formulaic, and mechanistic treatment of birthing people could give way to an open and rich engagement with birthing people and with births as expressions of unique bodies and minds, the deeply human experience of making human beings, and thereby worldmaking because, quite obviously, if people stopped giving birth, there would eventually be no more human beings.

Even within the context of the current hegemonic birth culture, many birthing people have been found to place great value on their ability to give birth physiologically and without biomedical interference (Davis-Floyd, 2022; Downe et al., 2018). Rather than receiving robust and effective support for so doing, many birthing people encounter naysayers, fearmongering, condescension, a myriad of obstacles, and incompatible contextual forces that undermine physiologic birth, let alone foster pleasurable birth experiences. This situation is compounded for Black, Brown, and Indigenous, and gender expansive birthing people by structural oppressions that further compromise their wellbeing, who, in addition to navigating the terrain of birth itself, must also navigate the politics and very real threats that they face in healthcare spaces (for multiple examples see Davis, 2019; Roberts, 2017; Howard, 2024; Oparah et al., 2016). In the relevant academic literature, the role of pleasure in birth has been handwaved largely as an irrelevant fluke and therefore seldom studied in earnest. As of this writing, no other biomedical, ethnographic, nor population-level studies have yet been published that examine the incidence or prevalence of pleasurable experiences associated with birth or potential relationships to birth outcomes. This book represents a first step in filling this gap, while attending to context from a critical intersectional feminist lens (Crenshaw, 1989).

The Historical Context of the Birth Culture in the United States

Today's hegemonic birth culture in the United States is rooted in Western European colonial and biomedical imperialism. Medical technologies for anesthesia originated in Europe in the mid-1800s and later spread to the United States and Canada (Wertz & Wertz, 1989; Rich, 1995). Ether and nitrous oxide were first used in medically attended births starting around 1842. When Queen Victoria of the United Kingdom was administered chloroform for her eighth birth in 1853 it triggered a wave of demand by upper-class White women in the West for birth anesthesia. In the latter half of the 1800s, anesthetized birth was part of a pronatalist, eugenic agenda. White upper-class women were encouraged to have more children to combat the declining birthrate and to alleviate racist concerns about demographic changes that would threaten the order of power (a concern that is just as relevant today). Anesthetized birth was promoted as a symbol of (White upper-class women's) liberation, seen as a feminist defiance of biblical notions of painful birth as punishment for original sin. First-wave White feminists were among the most vocal and vigorous promotors of anesthesia in birth (Wertz & Wertz, 1989; Rich, 1995).

The swell of demand for anesthetized birth in combination with deliveries via forceps by obstetricians, particularly by White upper-class women in the West, had been combined with the other social dynamics of the time to form foundational narratives of today's hegemonic birth culture, specifically in the United States but also beyond. The late 1800s and early 1900s heralded the expansion of the medicalization and the industrialization of the caring and healing professions (biomedicine, of course, but also, for example, teaching and psychology), and the expansion of capitalist thinking into service industries traditionally relegated to the realm of family or religious practice (Cahill, 2001; Martin, 2001). In concert with the spreading logics of industrialization, urbanization and modernization also played a role as those leaving their ancestral lands for the city tended to leave behind aspects of their traditional ways of living and knowing, assimilating into new, modernized identities aligned with White supremacy and xenophobia (Cahill, 2001; Martin, 2001). These trends collectively eroded and eradicated Indigenous and traditional birthways and modes of care across many groups, including European-rooted midwifery (and continue to do so across the globe today). Woman-led knowledge production and stewardship that had long been represented by ancestral birthways had also long been under assault as male-dominated allopathic medicine began expanding into birth care in the mid-1600s in Europe, both co-opting and displacing traditions of midwifery in the process. In the United States, the biomedical establishment leveraged sexist, classist, racist, and xenophobic rhetorics through strategic public campaigns aimed at discrediting and eliminating midwifery as a legitimate profession and to cement the dominance of allopathic obstetrics (Cooper Owens, 2017). These campaigns were largely successful. Hospitalized birth with allopathic doctors and nurses (for upper-class White women in the US at least) had become the norm by the 1940s.

Yet racialized and economically marginalized people had limited or no access to medically managed and anesthetized hospital birth, while at the same time their access to midwives and to other skilled traditional practitioners had been being actively and purposefully destroyed (Cooper Owens, 2017). The destruction of birth care access tracks with other horrific eugenic campaigns that had been raging during this time, including forced sterilizations and the experimentations of contraceptive technologies on Black, Brown, Indigenous, and low socioeconomic status White women and birthing people (Bruinius, 2007; Cooper Owens, 2017; Roberts, 2017). Painful, unsafe birth had been viewed as a useful deterrent to curb reproduction among groups thought by upper-class Whites to be "over-producing" or simply not worthy of existence (Bruinius, 2007; Cooper Owens, 2017, Cooper Owens & Fett, 2019; Davis, 2019). The current disparities and injustices in maternal and infant morbidity and mortality have roots in these lineages of oppression (Roberts, 2017; Davis, 2019).

"Twilight sleep" has become emblematic of the early stages of the medicalization of birth (Hairston, 1996; Leavitt, 1980, 2016; Rich, 1995; Thompson, 2019). Developed in 1906 by obstetricians Bernhardt Kronig and Karl Gauss in Germany, "twilight sleep" is a combined regimen of morphine for pain and scopolamine, a drug that causes amnesia. Twilight sleep, as had been promoted by first-wave feminists, particularly in New York, was branded as an idyllic birth in sophisticated, tranquil repose. This beautiful branding had successfully driven up the demand which had reached a fever-pitch during the 1910s. But beneath this dreamy euphemism hid a nightmarish reality. Scopolamine produced amnesia of the entire birth event but also caused disturbing behaviors in many laboring people. Mentally disoriented and in varying degrees of pain, laboring women under the influence of scopolamine often became unhinged, thrashing about wildly or violently. It then became standard protocol that birthing people were to be physically restrained (strapped to beds, latched into straitjackets, or even locked in cages) to prevent their biting, clawing, flailing around, striking, and otherwise harming their care providers or themselves. When mental normalcy eventually returned to the birthing person, however, no memories of the birth remained. Since no spouses, family, or other support persons had been allowed to be present, most birthing people were left unaware of just what had transpired in their twilight sleep—no memory, no pain, right?

Twilight sleep had largely gone out of fashion mostly among upper-class White women around World War I due to the difficulty of administering the medications, the strong concerns over the safety of the use of these medications and their negative effects on newborns, and nationalist sentiments against the use of German-born technologies (Rich, 1995). Eventually, multiple exposés were published in women's magazines during the 1950s, mostly by White mothers who'd been able to recall their horrific experiences of being under twilight sleep and by maternity nurses who had witnessed and had frequently administered twilight sleep births (Timeline, 2018). Even with the outcry that these publications had caused, twilight sleep continued to be used through the 1950s and, by some accounts, into the 1970s, particularly with People of Color. In fact, one of my interview participants, a Black woman from New York, reported having been born herself via a twilight sleep delivery her mother underwent in New York in 1961.

During the 1950s and 1960s, outside of the provision of twilight sleep, birth had taken on a typical pattern. A woman in labor was admitted to the hospital, put in a wheelchair, separated from all of her relatives, and taken to an examination room where her pubic hair was shaved, she was given a rectal enema and an antiseptic vaginal douche, and her dilation was manually checked (Davis-Floyd, 2022; Rich, 1995). She was then placed in a room, usually with many other women, to labor. She was refused food or drink. She may or may not have had a privacy screen, but she was typically left to labor alone, without a partner or support person other than an occasional visit from a nurse. She was typically forced to labor in the medical bed, on her back, and not permitted to freely move around the birthing space. Often, women in labor were tied to their hospital bed by their ankles and often by their wrists to restrain their movements. Occasionally, a doctor would, with or without warning or consent, manually check dilation by inserting their entire hand into the vagina and palpating the cervix, which is typically painful and greatly increases the risk of infection. The amniotic sac was ruptured, also increasing the risk of infection. Some doctors would also manually stretch the cervix, a maneuver that causes tremendous pain and potential injury. At crowning the mother would be dosed with ether to render her unconscious. Then the obstetrician would perform an episiotomy, which is an incision from the posterior edge of the vaginal opening through the perineum toward the anus, and then extract the baby with forceps. The baby would be slapped, cleaned, measured, and taken away to the nursery. It would typically be hours before the mother was allowed to meet her own child. This had all been done under the ideological aegis of what Robbie Davis-Floyd (2022) called "the industrial model of birth" (pp. 54–64). The doctors were the recipients of congratulations and, of course, ample payment.

During the 1970s, when the "technocratic model of birth" (Davis-Floyd, 2018, 2022) had ultimately cemented its hegemony in the United States, cesareans had rapidly begun to climb in rate, along with the accelerated and expanded use of many biomedical and technological interventions in medicalized birth management. The use of unsafe fetal X-rays was replaced by ultrasounds, which quickly became widespread. So too had electronic fetal monitoring, epidurals, spinal blocks, mechanical and pharmaceutical inductions and augmentations of labor, and a growing number of laboratory tests for both the pregnant person and the fetus, including screenings for congenital and genetic conditions.

Over time, some of the harmful practices that I've mentioned above have fallen out of favor, but that varies greatly depending on the location, practitioner, and institution. For example, forced pubic hair shaving, enemas, and restraints are now rare, although birthing people who are or have been serving time in US correctional facilities still experience being shackled during their labors and births (Ahrens, 2015). Episiotomies, once standard practice, are now waning in their use, yet they still happen, even against the expressed wishes of the birthing person (see Kimberly Turbin's case, Improving Birth, 2017; see also Tincello et al., 2003; Davis-Floyd, 2022, pp. 150–152). Whereas some methods fall away, other technologies continue to surge. Elective, meaning not medically indicated, cesareans are also on the rise, and their accompanying risks of placental disorders in subsequent pregnancies are now causing professionals to re-examine their approach to cesareans. Still, the cesarean rate in the US of 32% (CDC & National Center for Health Statistics, 2023, para. 1) is far above the standards that have been set by the WHO (2021), which recommends a cesarean rate of no higher than 15% (para. 1). Elective labor induction is currently surging. Labor inductions involve the use of biomedical technologies including devices and medications to dilate the cervix and to drive uterine contractions that ideally result in a vaginal birth, largely independent of the birthing person's innate physiology. Induction had once been uncommon unless medically indicated. However, with the 2018 publication of the ARRIVE trial, recommendations were swiftly adopted to push for inductions even for low-risk first pregnancies at 39 weeks, citing a reduction in cesarean rates in the induction group (Grobman et al., 2018). Studies are beginning to show that these shifts in practice have had mixed if not harmful results (Tassis et al., 2022, Nethery et al., 2023). The elective 39-week induction is the kinder, gentler version of the scheduled cesarean: fulfilling some of the same cultural, institutional, and economic preferences of healthcare systems, but with perhaps better optics than scheduled elective cesarean. Again, the otherwise organic, unruly, and mysterious nature of birth is brought to heel. The underlying ideologies of risk, control, and fear in birth settings drive the care, are easily weaponized, and impact racialized and otherwise historically marginalized people the most. To turn to Barbara Katz Rothman once more:

> The Biomedical Empire is still colonizing birth all over the world, as medically trained, nursing-based midwives are replacing what now get called traditional birth attendants. The US was unusual in trying to totally displace the midwives with physicians: Most countries brought midwifery under medical control. People trained in that medical model, having attended dozens of births, are brought in to replace the traditional birth attendants who have done hundreds, perhaps thousands of births in their communities. This is how the industry part of the Empire grows, and again, that means getting people to believe that their old ways were primitive, and that salvation comes with the new.
>
> *Katz Rothman, 2021, pp. 99*

It was in response to this overmedicalized birth management that the movement for natural birth had first emerged in the late 1960s. Grantly Dick-Read in the 1940s in England, Ferdinand Lamaze in the 1950s in France, and Robert Bradley in 1965 in the United States, all White male allopathic medical doctors, each published still widely read books on their differing approaches to naturally reducing pain during birth (Rich, 1995, p. 173). Drawing on these influences, the natural birth movement in the United States (1950s and 1960s) grew among largely coastal, college-educated, counter-cultural, alternative lifestyle types, often termed "hippies," who were largely White middle and upper class. "The Farm" in Summertown, Tennessee is one famous example (see Ina May Gaskin's three also still widely read books). Indeed, the works of Ina May Gaskin, who is still considered by many to be the most famous midwife in the world, remain major resources among those who are pursuing de-medicalized birth experiences (Gaskin, 2008; 2010; 2011).

The Black and Brown feminist movements for reproductive and birth justice, and the movement for the decolonization of birth (which is considered by some to be part of the origins of the third and fourth waves of feminism), to varying degrees engage in push-back against the technocratic and medicalized paradigms of birth while reclaiming and restoring traditional birth care paradigms in resistance to overmedicalization, obstetric racism, and obstetric violence. The reproductive justice movement was most visibly launched and lead by Black feminists during the 1970s in counter to the White second-wave feminist movements that focused on the pro-life/pro-choice debates and on contraception access (especially targeting teens) but had failed to address the major human rights issues facing Black and Brown people—forced contraception or sterilization, medical experimentation, poverty, criminalization, economic exploitation, medical neglect, coercion, and violence (Oparah et al., 2016). According to Ross and Solinger (2017),

> Reproductive justice goes beyond the pro-choice/pro-life debate and has three primary principles: (1) the right *not* to have a child; (2) the right to *have* a child; (3) the right to *parent* children in safe and healthy environments. In addition, reproductive justice demands sexual autonomy and gender freedom for every human being.
>
> *Ross and Solinger, 2017, p. 9, emphases in original*

This crisp definition of reproductive justice, however, does not address *how to have a child, where, and with whom.* As such, this definition preserves something of an exception around birth, placing birth somewhere just beyond its scope. Birth itself was often absent from early works for reproductive rights. Birth justice emerged more recently as a movement, led by Black and Brown women, roughly during the early 2010s, to address the intersectional oppressions that had been and still are facing birthing People of Color. Black and Brown birthworkers, as ever, are facing down obstetric racism, overmedicalization, and obstetric violence, and are creating strategies and responses to protect birthing people from harm within and outside of medicalized spaces. These strategies include building doula collectives, community-based midwifery practices, autonomous birth centers, and increasing access to home birth, within and beyond their legality (Foster-McCray, 2024). Birth justice activists currently challenge the racist, classist, ableist, and cisheteronormative frames that have been and still are dominant in the natural birth movement and instead center birth as a nexus of social justice transformation.

Some connect the work of early "natural" or "physiological" birth advocates to White supremacist, sexist, patriarchal, and racist pronatalist agendas that drove the demand for anesthetized birth in the late 1800s up to the mid-1900s by upper-class White women. Premier among them were Grantley Dick-Read's (1942/2004) *Childbirth Without Fear*, for example, and the work of Ferdinand Lamaze (popularized in the 1950s), Robert Bradley's (1965/2008) *Husband-Coached Childbirth*, and Michel Odent's (1987, 1991, 2007, 2021) long career of work. I acknowledge this critique; however, I also see narrative through-lines connecting these early natural birth advocates' work with longstanding knowledge grounded in midwifery and many traditional birthways. These White male practitioners of Western allopathic medicine were not the original and ultimate source of the appropriated birth knowledge that made them world-famous. That wisdom came from a long lineage of women, midwives, and birthworkers stretching back into time immemorial (see Ehrenreich & English, 2010; Trevathan, 2010). These are traditionally women's wisdoms, with rich cultural differences and deep ancestral roots all over the world. I do, however, give these White male "natural" birth advocates credit for promoting ways of thinking about birth that defied hegemonic biomedicalization; some of the ideas they espoused are found in the shared terrains of birth activism and birth justice.

The terrain of birth activism and birth justice is vast and deserves its own book, or several. But to sketch it briefly herein, the movement that is challenging the present hegemonic and technocratic birth culture, and thereby the Biomedical Empire, starts with birthing people themselves, their families, their support persons, and their partners in their politics of care. Doulas of many kinds, childbirth educators from a variety of disciplines, and of course midwives of many stripes have long led this space (Salinas et al., 2022). It also includes rebellious allopathic doctors, osteopathic doctors, and obstetricians critical of the overmedicalization of birth and iatrogenic birth harm (for multiple examples of such criticisms written by obstetricians themselves, see *Obstetricians Speak: On Training, Practice, Fear, and Transformation* by Davis-Floyd & Premkumar, 2023c; for an in-depth discussion of iatrogenic birth harms, see Liese et al., 2021). Many birth-focused practitioners also participate. This movement also includes many organizations working to improve birth experiences, within and beyond the biomedical space, including legal professionals and policymakers. It includes efforts to de-medicalize birth by promoting physiological, "natural," ecstatic, orgasmic, and/or hypnobirthing. It also includes movements for community birth in autonomous birth centers or in homes, including professional midwife-assisted, traditional-midwife assisted, or even unassisted "free birth." Further, movements to decolonize birth among Indigenous communities and racialized folks continue to challenge colonized ways of knowing about and giving birth, and the care of birthing people.

The thematic through-lines permeate the second-wave feminist movements for bodily autonomy, pleasure, sexual liberation, and gender equality. They also are palpable in the current reproductive and birth justice movements (and in the third and fourth-wave feminisms). And still, racial and classist fissures remain salient in the outgrowths of the natural birth movement. More recently, some White homebirth activists have shed the "crunchy" radical, hippie, feminist image of the natural birth movement and of its politics to better align with classist and racist neoliberal respectability politics—that good citizen-consumers deserve the market choice to choose homebirth and midwifery care—with some success (Craven, 2010). The White neoliberal capitalist infiltration and cooptation of social movements is nothing new. Similar dynamics have been called out among those struggling for 2SLGBTQQAI+ (two-spirit, lesbian, gay, bisexual, transgender, queer, questioning, asexual, intersex) justice (Vaid, 2012). Movements for 2SLGBTQQAI+ reproductive and family-building rights, including gender-expansive birthways (which are entwined with third and fourth-wave feminisms), are also engaging critically and strategically with the medicalization of births. Queer birthing people continue to grapple with how biomedicalization in the process of family-building is experienced, internalized, and transformed into resistance against engrained White supremacy and cisheteropatriarchy, particularly within medicalized birth spaces (Light et al., 2014).

Foreseeably, my emphasis on pleasure in the reproductive experience is predictably juicy fodder for the misogynist, regressive "keep 'em barefoot and pregnant in the kitchen" contingent. A real danger lies in the cooptation of my arguments for the liberation of joy and pleasure in birth, which could be read as an endorsement of pronatalist agendas. I'm not alone in sensing this tension. As Katz Rothman put it in her analysis of the "Biomedical Empire": "one ongoing concern is how to wrest the critique of biomedicine from right wing populism" (p. 13). I am not interested in my work being misconstrued as evidence for eugenic-rooted, racist, pronatalist agendas. Rather, I am interested in childbearers' liberation from the enforced reproductive and maternal misery perpetuated in the US and around the world. I'm reminded of two interlocutors' accounts:

> I really had to take over and claim—and reclaim—my agency. And I think had I not, it [birth] wouldn't have been a pleasurable experience by any means.
>
> *Cande*

> I rewired my brain for thinking about labor in a pleasurable way. And that and in doing so, you know, reclaimed, like power that was taken from me in the first two births.
>
> *Aleks*

In reclaiming power in ways that transcend generations, nations, racialization, genders, and social locations, there is resistance to hegemonic medicalized pain-and-fear-centric birth culture, and further, biomedical empire. This resistance sings in many voices. It condemns over-medicalization, obstetric violence, obstetric racism, sexual and gendered violence, colonization, and the disruption of traditional birthways. So too, pleasure sings. Pleasure sings in defiance. Let us listen to that song now. I'll turn up the volume.

References

Ahrens, D. (2015). Incarcerated childbirth and broader birth control: Autonomy, regulation, and the state. *Missouri Law Review*, *80*(1), 1–51. https://scholarship.law.missouri.edu/mlr/vol80/iss1/5

Bradley, R. A. (2008). *Husband-coached childbirth: The Bradley method of natural childbirth*. Bantam. (Original work published 1965)

Bruinius, H. (2007). *Better for all the world: The secret history of forced sterilization and America's quest for racial purity*. Vintage.

Cahill, H. A. (2001). Male appropriation and medicalization of childbirth: An historical analysis. *Journal of Advanced Nursing*, *33*, 334–342. https://doi.org/10.1046/j.1365-2648.2001.01669.x

CDC & National Center for Health Statistics (2023). *Births – Method of delivery*. FastStats Homepage. www.cdc.gov/nchs/fastats/delivery.htm

Cooper Owens, D. (2017). *Medical bondage: Race, gender, and the origins of American gynecology*. University of Georgia Press.

Cooper Owens, D., & Fett, S. M. (2019). Black maternal and infant health: Historical legacies of slavery. *American Journal of Public Health*, *109*(10), 1342–1345. https://doi.org/10.2105/AJPH.2019.305243

Craven, C. (2010). *Pushing for midwives: Homebirth mothers and the reproductive rights movement*. Temple University Press.

Crenshaw, K. (1989). Demarginalizing the intersection of race and sex: A Black feminist critique of antidiscrimination doctrine, feminist theory and antiracist politics. *University of Chicago Legal Forum*, *1989*(1), 139–167. http://chicagounbound.uchicago.edu/uclf/vol1989/iss1/8

Creedy, D. K., Shochet, I. M., & Horsfall, J. (2000). Childbirth and the development of acute trauma symptoms: Incidence and contributing factors. *Birth*, *27*(2), 104–111. https://doi.org/10.1046/j.1523-536x.2000.00104.x

Davis, D. A. (2019). Obstetric racism: The racial politics of pregnancy, labor, and birthing. *Medical Anthropology*, *38*(7), 560–573. https://doi.org/10.1080/01459740.2018.1549389

Davis-Floyd, R. (2003). *Birth as an American rite of passage: With a new preface*. University of California Press.

Davis-Floyd, R. (2018). *Ways of knowing about birth: Mothers, midwives, medicine, and birth activism*. Waveland Press.

Davis-Floyd, R. (2022). *Birth as an American rite of passage* (3rd ed.). Routledge.

Davis-Floyd, R., & Premkumar, A. (Eds.). (2023a). *Cognition, risk, and responsibility in obstetrics: Anthropological analyses and critiques of obstetricians' practices*: The anthropology of obstetrics and obstetricians—Volume II. Berghahn Books.

Davis-Floyd, R., & Premkumar, A. (Eds.). (2023b). *Obstetric violence and systemic disparities: Can obstetrics be humanized and decolonized?* The anthropology of obstetrics and obstetricians—Volume III. Berghahn Books.

Davis-Floyd, R., & Premkumar, A. (Eds.). (2023c). *Obstetricians speak: On training, practice, fear, and transformation: The anthropology of obstetrics and obstetricians—Volume I*. Berghahn Books.

Delaporte, M. (2018). Curse to co-creation: Religious models of labour pain. *Journal of the Motherhood Initiative for Research and Community Involvement*, *9*(2) 103–113. https://jarm.journals.yorku.ca/index.php/jarm/article/view/40548

Dick-Read, G. (2004). *Childbirth without fear: The principles and practice of natural childbirth*. Pinter & Martin (Original work published 1942).

Downe, S., Finlayson, K., Oladapo, O., Bonet, M., & Gülmezoglu, A. M. (2018). What matters to women during childbirth: A systematic qualitative review. *PLOS ONE*, *13*(4), e0194906. https://doi.org/10.1371/journal.pone.0194906

Ehrenreich B., & English D. (2010). *Witches, midwives, and nurses: A History of women healers* (2nd ed.). The Free Press.

Foster-McCray, A. (2024, November 20–23). *Outside the warehouse of risk: Caesarean violence, antiblackness, and illegal home birth culture in urban and rural Georgia, USA* [Conference Presentation]. American Anthropological Association Annual Meeting, Tampa, FL, USA.

Gaskin, I. M. (2008). *Ina May's guide to childbirth: Updated with new material*. Bantam.

Gaskin, I. M. (2010). *Spiritual midwifery*. Book Publishing Company.

Gaskin, I. M. (2011). *Birth matters: A midwife's manifesta*. Seven Stories Press.

Geissbuehler, V., & Eberhard, J. (2002). Fear of childbirth during pregnancy: A study of more than 8000 pregnant women. *Journal of Psychosomatic Obstetrics & Gynecology*, *23*(4), 229–235. https://doi.org/10.3109/01674820209074677

Grobman, W. A., Rice, M. M., Reddy, U. M., Tita, A. T., Silver, R. M., Mallett, G., ... & Macones, G. A. (2018). Labor induction versus expectant management in low-risk nulliparous women. *New England Journal of Medicine*, *379*(6), 513–523.

Hairston, A. H. (1996). The debate over twilight sleep: Women influencing their medicine. *Journal of Women's Health*, *5*(5), 489–499. https://doi.org/10.1089/jwh.1996.5.489

Hofberg, K., & Brockington, I. F. (2000). Tokophobia: An unreasoning dread of childbirth. *The British Journal of Psychiatry*, *176*(1), 83–85. https://doi.org/10.1192/bjp.176.1.83

Hogg, M. A., Abrams, D., & Martin, G. N. (2010). Social cognition and attitudes. In G. N. Martin, N. R. Carlson, & W. Buskist (Eds.), *Psychology* (pp. 646–677). Pearson Education.

Howard, G. E. (2024). *The pregnancy police: Conceiving crime, arresting personhood* (Vol. 10). University of California Press.

Improving Childbirth. (2017). *Kimberly Turbin's forced episiotomy case: The resolution*. https://improvingbirth.org/2017/03/kimberlys-case-the-resolution/

Katz Rothman, B. (2021). *The Biomedical empire: Lessons learned from the COVID-19 pandemic*. Stanford University Press.

Leachman, A. (2017). How media promote fear around childbirth. In A. Luce, V. Hundley, & E. Van Teijlingen (Eds.). *Midwifery, childbirth and the media* (pp. 61–77). Springer International.

Leavitt, J. W. (1980). Birthing and anesthesia: The debate over twilight sleep. *Signs: Journal of Women in Culture and Society*, 6(1). https://doi.org/10.1086/493783

Leavitt, J. W. (2016). *Brought to bed: Childbearing in America, 1750–1950.* Oxford University Press.

Liese K., Davis-Floyd R., Stewart K., & Cheyney, M. (2021). Obstetric iatrogenesis in the United States: The spectrum of unintentional harm, disrespect, violence, and abuse. *Anthropology & Medicine*, *28*(2), 1–17. https://doi.org/10.1080/13648470.2021.1938510

Light, A. D., Obedin-Maliver, J., Sevelius, J. M., & Kerns, J. L. (2014). Transgender men who experienced pregnancy after female-to-male gender transitioning. *Obstetrics & Gynecology*, *124*(6), 1120–1127. https://doi.org/10.1097/aog.0000000000000540

Martin, E. (2001). *The woman in the body: A cultural analysis of reproduction.* Beacon Press.

Nethery, E., Levy, B., McLean, K., Sitcov, K., & Souter, V. L. (2023). Effects of the ARRIVE (A randomized trial of induction versus expectant management) trial on elective induction and obstetric outcomes in term nulliparous patients. *Obstetrics and Gynecology*, *142*(2), 242–250. https://doi.org/10.1097/AOG.0000000000005217

Odent, M. (1987). The fetus ejection reflex. *Birth: Issues in Perinatal Care*, *14*(2), 104–105. https://doi.org/10.1111/j.1523-536X.1987.tb01463.x

Odent, M. (1991). Fear of death during labour. *Journal of Reproductive and Infant Psychology*, *9*(1), 43–47. https://doi.org/10.1080/02646839108403655

Odent, M. (2007). *Birth and breastfeeding: Rediscovering the needs of women during pregnancy and childbirth.* Clairview Books.

Odent, M. (2021). Is labor a complication of socialized birth? In *Midwifery Today*. www.midwiferytoday.com/mt-articles/is-labor-a-complication-of-socialized-birth/

Oparah, J. C., & Black Women Birthing Justice. (2016). Beyond coersion and malign neglect: Black women and the struggle for birth justice, introduction. In J. C. Oparah & A. D. Bonaparte (Eds.), *Birthing justice: Black women, pregnancy, and childbirth.* Routledge.

Rich, A. (1995). *Of woman born.* W. W. Norton.

Roberts, D. (2017). *Killing the black body: Race, reproduction, and the meaning of liberty.* Vintage.

Ross, L., & Solinger, R. (2017). *Reproductive justice: An introduction.* University of California Press.

Salinas, J. L., Salinas, M., & Kahn, M. (2022). Doulas, racism, and Whiteness: How birth support workers process advocacy towards women of color. *Societies*, *12*(1), 19. https://doi.org/10.3390/soc12010019

Sheen, K., & Slade, P. (2018). Examining the content and moderators of women's fears for giving birth: A meta-synthesis. *Journal of Clinical Nursing*, *27*(13–14), 2523–2535. https://doi.org/10.1111/jocn.14219

Tassis, B. M. G., Ruggiero, M., Ronchi, A., Ramezzana, I. G., Bischetti, G., Iurlaro, E., D'Ambrosi, F., Ciralli, F., Mosca, F., & Ferrazzi, E. M. (2022). An hypothetical external validation of the ARRIVE trial in a European academic hospital. *Journal of Maternal-Fetal & Neonatal Medicine: The Official Journal of the European Association of Perinatal Medicine, the Federation of Asia and Oceania Perinatal Societies, the International Society of Perinatal Obstetricians*, *35*(22), 4291–4298. https://doi.org/10.1080/14767058.2020.1849108

Thompson, L. M. (2019). The politics of female pain: Women's citizenship, twilight sleep and the early birth control movement. *Medical Humanities*, *45*(1), 67–74. http://doi.org/10.1136/medhum-2017-011419

Timeline. (2018). *"Twilight sleep" offered the promise of painless birth—but at what cost? How a Ladies' Home Journal expose ended one of the most controversial birthing techniques*. Retrieved January 22, 2023, from https://timeline.com/twilight-sleep-pregnancy-child-birth-womens-health-video-history-decf81e729f1

Tincello, D. G., Williams, A., Fowler, G. E., Adams, E. J., Richmond, D. H., & Alfirevic, Z. (2003). Differences in episiotomy technique between midwives and doctors. *BJOG: An International Journal of Obstetrics & Gynaecology*, *110*(12), 1041–1044. https://doi.org/10.1016/S1470-0328(03)03930-2

Trevathan, W. (2010). *Ancient bodies, modern lives: How evolution has shaped women's health*. Oxford University Press.

Vaid, U. (2012). *Irresistible revolution: Confronting race, class and the assumptions of lesbian, gay, bisexual, and transgender politics*. Magnus Books.

Wertz, R. W., & Wertz, D. C. (1989). *Lying-in: A history of childbirth in America*. Yale University Press.

Wigert, H., Nilsson, C., Dencker, A., Begley, C., Jangsten, E., Sparud-Lundin, C., Mollberg, M., & Patel, H. (2020). Women's experiences of fear of childbirth: A metasynthesis of qualitative studies. International Journal of Qualitative Studies on Health and Wellbeing, *15*(1), 1704484. https://doi.org/10.1080/17482631.2019.1704484

World Health Organization. (2021). *WHO Statement on caesarean section rates*. www.who.int/news-room/questions-and-answers/item/who-statement-on-caesarean-section-rates-frequently-asked-questions

2

BIRTH PLEASURE EXPERIENCES AND PERCEPTIONS

This chapter explores my study participants' experiences of birth pleasure, first attending to their perceptions of their own experiences, then focusing in on the typology of birth pleasure that emerged through my qualitative analyses in its five apparent aspects: emotional, mental, physical, sexual, and spiritual. While these types of pleasure are conceptualized separately in this typology for the sake of analysis, this conceptualization is necessarily fraught. In most interview participants' experiences (and mine), many aspects of pleasure co-arose as layered and entwined, alongside pain or in its absence. For example, an emotion might generate physical sensations or vice versa. A mental state, such as a euphoric altered state of consciousness, shifts the perceptions of physical sensations or emotions. Emotions can color the interpretation of physical sensations, thereby making them more or less pleasurable, painful, banal, or erotic. I have not meant, by having parsed out a typology of pleasure, to be constraining but rather to create access for my readers to more nuanced understandings of my study participants' birth experiences within these data and potentially beyond them.

Perceptions of Experiences of Birth Pleasure

One thematic element that emerged in four of the interviews but had felt simultaneously a sidenote and a key finding was how these pleasurable experiences had been perceived by the study participants. Because these

DOI: 10.4324/9781003499428-3

topics are so rarely discussed, many participants had agreed to participate in this study because it had been a welcome opportunity to discuss their birth experiences. For many, our interviews had been first time that they had granted any real validity to their birth pleasure experiences.

During our interview, Romi shared a desire to talk through her experience, having felt that there had not been enough space to discuss pleasure in birth during ordinary postpartum conversations:

> I feel like I've wanted to talk about it, and I have with some people, but it can be hard to talk about, because most women don't have this experience. So first of all, you know, you don't want to like, you don't want to sort of gloat to other women who have had kind of traumatic experiences, because a lot of women have. And so, it's kind of awkward to talk about. And it's also a bit of an isolating experience, because it seems so rare. And so, I've had this experience, I've been trying to find a place to put it and to talk about it.

Pearl had also kept her pleasurable birth experiences to herself. During our interview, she told me:

> Yeah, postpartum there were a lot of like birth groups that I went to that was like, facilitated by the midwives. So, you could talk about your experience. And I remember feeling the majority of people stories were traumatic, in different ways. And so, I wanted to, while I could express my story, I wanted to give space for them, you know, and so I felt like I always held back quite a bit and being like, "I had this amazing blah blah blah," you know, when they're like in tears, because they, you know, still have tears that are challenging and they weren't able to make decisions, or whatever. So, I do definitely feel like I've held back in circles, where people are talking about their birth story, and wanting to make space for that more, even though I deserve space and pleasure, deserves space. It—I have this sense of like, I don't want to be like "Well, my birth experience was," you know [Laughs] … I definitely would feel like hesitant to go in depth about it. If it weren't, like consciously asked about, you know?

When Melissa had shared about her pleasurable birth experiences with others, the sense that she got was that she was being viewed as special, "a unicorn," and that her sharing of her birth experience was perhaps interesting but of little real-life relevance to the listener. During our interview, she shared:

> I mean, they hear my story, and I guess it's a good one. And they seem intrigued and interested, maybe hopeful to have a similar experience, but they almost always say, "Oh, you're strong, I could never do that." And I'm like, "I'm not, I'm not—I'm just a regular person." It's, it's almost like I say, it's like a unicorn like, like women who experience pleasure in birth or have this, come out of it with this, like, positive "I want to do it again and again," attitude, it's like, something that exists out there, but that can't be for me.

Dalisay had also minimized the importance of her own pleasurable birth experience, particularly her spiritual vision and the euphoria, which she had filed way in the back of her mind along with the trauma of her first birth experience. In her words:

> When I had my firstborn, and then that—I had that same feeling, the same sensation, the same everything and the same sort of out of body experience, and then verbalizing something that was so irrational, and only me, only I can understand [laughs] and, and, and no one else would know what I'm talking about. You know, it was really bizarre. And, you know, and it happens in—within a split second, until my rational mind tells me "This is not true, this is not real." And then I have to go back into like reality of like, "Well, maybe that's just—" you know, whatever, maybe some fantasies, maybe some other something, you know, unexplainable, but, you know, but that's not real. So. So anyway, that, you know, that was my birth experience with my son. And I haven't had any experiences like that ever again … So I think I pushed it aside. After that experience, and I never really talked about it again. I don't even remember if I mentioned that to my husband. When it happened, I don't think I did. And even if I did, I don't think he would have put a lot of meaning to it. So, I think after that happened, I kind of pushed it aside, like … the rational mind "Maybe that was just because of the drugs or the rush of hormones" or "I was tired." So, I really did not give meaning to it either. Until you started talking about your study—then, that's when it was kind of like, "Oh!" It clicked. Maybe I had a pleasurable birth experience. Because this whole time I was thinking that that was not pleasurable, you know? My first birth was so painful and so traumatic. And the use of these machineries for the childbirth—I'd rather forget about all that. And, and I didn't really want to think about that trauma. That one moment of pleasure just got filed away as part of that whole process of, like, "painful, horrible, done," you know? I'm so glad that I came out of that in one piece, and my child came out of that in one piece.

Dalisay contacted me asking to participate in this study after hearing me speak about the topic of birth pleasure, which prompted her to reconsider her experiences from a different perspective. As she described during our interview:

> So, I never really thought of it until you started talking about how women can actually have pleasurable birth experiences! And not just, you know—not just any normal pleasure, but it's actually something profound that happens to them. You know, whether it's having an orgasm or some other something. And so, when you were explaining these things, at first, I was thinking of orgasm only. Like, pleasure as in my feeling, you know, as pleasure as in sexual pleasure. But, as I thought of it, I'm like, "You know, to me, *that was pleasure*," you know, the pleasure of being in that realm that I cannot explain—*that was pleasure*. And being in a space that I could never replicate again was pleasure. In a space where it just happened so spontaneously, and it happened without me willing it to happen, was pleasure ... That [birth] was 19 or 18 years ago ... That experience was so vivid. I mean a lot of the details of that childbirth was a little—very blurry to me now. But that one moment of that one experience is still so vivid to me. And I don't think I'll ever forget that. It is an experience that I think I can hold on to for the rest of my life ... pleasure meaning happiness, and euphoria, and all of these other things.

Debbie raised her hand to participate in this study, in part because she had never talked about her lustful postpartum experience with anyone else:

> Yeah. I never talked to anybody about it ... That's one of the reasons I was so excited to talk to you, you know? Someone else. Someone else might, you know, know why. I'm not—not necessarily the only person. I'm not necessarily that weird.

In terms of the "why," Debbie offered the following hypothesis for why this lustful postpartum experience might have happened: "That [experience of birth] will bond you two together as parents during the upcoming very difficult time. Right? Maybe there's a physiological purpose for that." Unfortunately, I had not been able to answer her question of "why" with this study alone. But her hypothesis is compelling and is biologically plausible. In the quest to expand the ways in which birth experiences are understood and thereby made better, birth pleasure experiences, even relatively unusual ones like Debbie's, matter—especially those experiences that are rendered invisible, hidden, shamed, or rationalized away as being anomalies rather than being taken seriously. None of my participants had explicitly reported having informed their care providers or their partners about the pleasure that they had experienced during their births. These pleasurable birthing experiences might have been visible to their care providers, but my guess is that they were not. Someday, if I could get charts (from whatever practitioner might be present, if any) and see if pleasure is ever mentioned, I would love to do that study. Has pleasure ever been documented in a birthing person's chart? If one were to do a study based on records alone, what would be there about pleasure? My sense is very little or nothing at all. But this work remains to, and should, be done. In the meantime, I generally saw a hesitancy to name or discuss these kinds of pleasurable birth experiences with others among my interview participants.

A Typology of Birth Pleasure

All 23 interview participants reported having experienced both emotional and mental pleasure during their births (100%). Twenty-one participants reported having experienced physical pleasure (91%), held as distinct from sexual pleasure. Eleven participants discussed what I coded as "spiritual pleasure," because they had used spiritual concepts to articulate their pleasurable experiences (48%). Lastly, eight interview participants described the pleasure that they had experienced during their births as having been sexual in some way (35%). For an overview of each participant and the types of pleasure they had experienced during their births, see Table 2.1. Also see Figure 2.1 which offers a visual depiction of the Birth Pleasure-Pain Spectra.

I would also like to draw my readers' attention to my summaries of the participants' demographics that I've placed in the Appendix to this book. Also see Tables 2.2, 2.3, and 2.4, which respectively summarize the study participants' racial and ethnic identities, gender and sexual orientations, and class markers. Also, I have included a chart with brief narrative snapshots of each participant's identities and birth experiences in Appendix B. Please note that I've presented as much detailed information as my study participants offered, some of whom had specified many details about their racial and ancestral identities, while others had simply indicated a broad racial category (White, or Black/African American, for example). Some interview participants declined to provide certain information, such as their income. Some interview participants were clear about certain details, such as where they were when they were giving birth (particularly those who had moved since the birth), and others left that information vague, so I've specified these details wherever possible.

TABLE 2.1 The Birth Pleasure-Pain Spectra: An Overview of the Study Participants' Experiences

Pseudonym	*Birth Pleasure-Pain Spectra*						
	Birth Pleasure Typology					*Pain-free Birth*[a]	
	Emotional	*Mental*	*Physical*	*Sexual*	*Spiritual*	*Whole*	*In part*
Aleks	*	*	*	*			*
Araceli	*	*	*		*	*	
Bree	*	*	*			*	
Callie	*	*	*		*		
Callisto	*	*	*				*
Cande	*	*	*	*			*
Chandra	*	*	*			*	
Dalisay	*	*	*		*		
Debbie	*	*	*	*			
Fabia	*	*	*			*	
Malika	*	*					
Marion	*	*	*	*			*
Melissa	*	*			*		
Nava	*	*	*	*	*	*	
Pearl	*	*	*	*			
Raquel	*	*	*				*[b]
Romi	*	*	*		*		
Sankofa	*	*	*		*		
Semiramis	*	*	*		*		
Skylar	*	*	*		*	*	
Theia	*	*	*			*	
Venus	*	*	*	*	*		
Veronica	*	*	*	*	*		
Total[c]	23	23	21	8	11	7	5
Percent	100%	100%	91%	35%	48%	30%	22%

Notes:

[a] Pain-free physiological birth without analgesia

[b] Reported pain-free experience without analgesia for most of induced labor, increased pain with Pitocin administration, and received an epidural due to concerns over fetal heart tones. Shortly thereafter she was found to be complete (10cm) and instructed to push.

[c] This table summarizes the number of interview participants who reported ever having experienced the types of birth pleasure or pain-free birth delineated in the Birth Pleasure-Pain Spectra (not the number of pleasurable birth experiences, which might be more than one for the same birthing person).

Emotional Pleasure

Feeling good in the context of birth included many shades of emotion. I coded descriptions of any emotional state they emphasized as pleasurable or positive, such as joy, love, peace, or excitement as *emotional pleasure.*

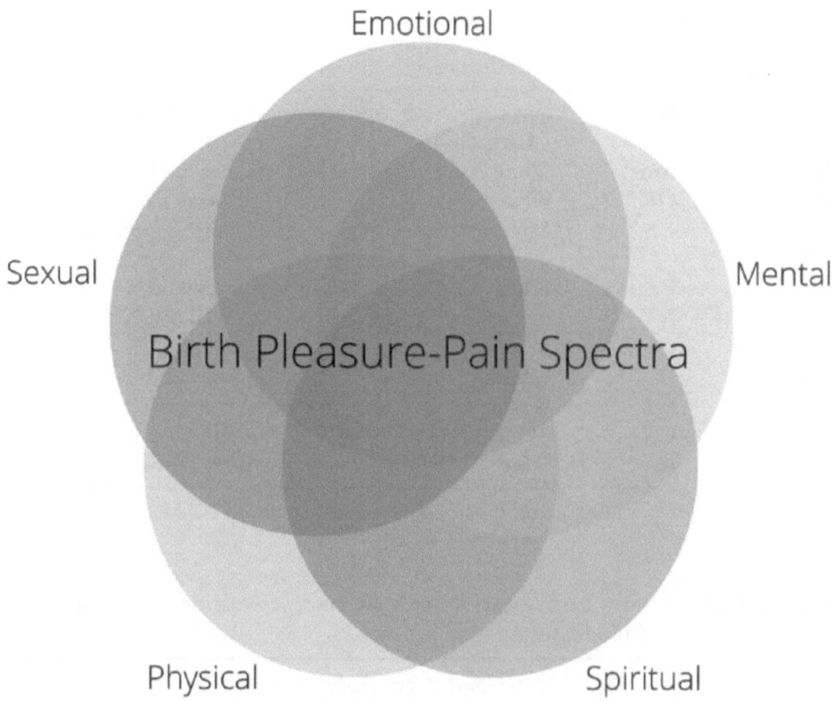

FIGURE 2.1 The Birth Pleasure-Pain Spectra.

TABLE 2.2 The Study Participants' Demographics: Their Locations, Races/Ethnicities, and Their Places of Origin

Pseudonym	*Location*	*Race/Ethnicity*	*Origin*
Aleks	MD	White Russian Armenian	Azerbaijan
Araceli	CA	Latina Mexican-American Binational	Mexico City, MX
Bree	UT	Asian/Pacific Islander Vietnamese	Vietnam
Callie	NY	Black/African American	Harbor City, CA
Callisto	IL	Black/African American	Syracuse, NY
Cande	NY	Latine Mexican Mestize	Santa Barbara, CA
Chandra	CA	Black/African American	Brooklyn, NY
Dalisay	CA	Asian/Pacific Islander Filipina	Philippines
Debbie	CO	White	Unstated
Fabia	England	White Spaniard	Avila, Spain
Malika	CA	Black/African American	Berkeley, CA
Marion	CA	White Dutch	Calistoga, CA

(*Continued*)

TABLE 2.2 (Continued)

Pseudonym	*Location*	*Race/Ethnicity*	*Origin*
Melissa	NY	Black/African American + Latina	Brooklyn, NY
Nava	Israel	White Ashkenazi Israeli Jew	White Plains, NY
Pearl	OR	White	Worcester, MA
Raquel	CA	Asian/Pacific Islander Chinese	Washington state
Romi	CA	White-passing Moroccan Jew	Oakland, CA
Sankofa	NY	Black/African American	Yonkers, NY
Semiramis	CA	Arab + European	Melrose, MA
Skylar	IA	White	Unstated
Theia	WI	White	Eau Claire, WI
Venus	CA	White	San Diego, CA
Veronica	IA	White	Okinawa, Japan

Note: Location abbreviations refer to states in the United States; MX is Mexico.

TABLE 2.3 The Study Participants' Demographics: Sexualities, Genders, and Relationship Statuses

Pseudonym	*Sexuality, Gender, and Relationship*		
	Gender	*Sexual Orientation*[a]	*Relationship Status*
Aleks	Agender Queer	L	Married Open
Araceli	Cis/Woman	H	Married Exclusive
Bree	Cis/Woman	H	Married Exclusive
Callie	Cis/Woman	H	Married Exclusive
Callisto	Cis/Woman	H	Married Exclusive
Cande	Non-binary	Q	Married Exclusive
Chandra	Cis/Woman	H	Single
Dalisay	Cis/Woman	H	Married Exclusive
Debbie	Cis/Woman	H	Married Exclusive
Fabia	Cis/Woman	Hm	Married Exclusive
Malika	Cis/Woman	H	Married Exclusive
Marion	Cis/Woman	H	Married Exclusive
Melissa	Cis/Woman	H	Married Exclusive
Nava	Cis/Woman	H	Married Exclusive
Pearl	Cis/Woman	Bi	Married Exclusive
Raquel	Cis/Woman	H	Married Exclusive
Romi	Cis/Woman	H	Married Exclusive
Sankofa	Cis/Woman	Bi	Married Open
Semiramis	Womxn	Q	Single
Skylar	Cis/Woman	H	Married Exclusive
Theia	Cis/Woman	L	Single

TABLE 2.3 (Continued)

Pseudonym	*Sexuality, Gender, and Relationship*		
	Gender	*Sexual Orientation*[a]	*Relationship Status*
Venus	Cis/Woman	H/Bi (prior)	Married Exclusive
Veronica	Cis/Woman	H	Married Exclusive

Note: [a] Sexual orientation abbreviations meanings:

H	Heterosexual
Hm	Mostly Heterosexual
Bi	Bisexual
Q	Queer
L	Lesbian

TABLE 2.4 The Study Participants' Demographics: Socioeconomic Statuses and Class Factors

Pseud.	*Socioeconomic Status and Class Factors*					
	Annual Income US$	*Family Size*	*Housing*	*Occupation*	*Insurancea*	*Education*[b]
Aleks	$90,000	6	Own	Professor, author	P/EB	6
Araceli	$90,000	4	Rent	Ed. researcher	P/EB	6
Bree	$100,000	3	Rent	Business partner	None	4
Callie	$200,000	3	Rent	Professor, academic	P/EB	6
Callisto	$90,000	3	Own	Doula	P/EB	6
Cande	$106,000	3	Own	Consult. researcher	P/EB	6
Chandra	$64,000	3	Own	Doula, trainer	P/EB	6
Dalisay	$250,000	4	Own	Government	P/EB	6
Debbie	Med-High*	4	Own	Teaching/ nursing	P/EB	6
Fabia	$99,000	4	Own	Midwife	Public	5
Malika	$20,000	3	Unhoused	Poet	Public	5
Marion	$55,000	4	Rent	Stay-at-home mother	P/EB	4
Melissa	$120,000	4	Rent/ Own	Doula	P/EB	4
Nava	$18,000	3	Rent/ Own	Student, writing	Public	6

(*Continued*)

TABLE 2.4 (Continued)

Pseud.	*Socioeconomic Status and Class Factors*					
	Annual Income US$	*Family Size*	*Housing*	*Occupation*	*Insurancea*	*Education*[b]
Pearl	$38,000	3	Own	Admin, counselor	Public	6
Raquel	$300,000	3	Rent	Designer	P/EB	6
Romi	$100,000	4	Own	Therapist	P/EB	6
Sankofa	$60,000	7	Own	Midwife	P/EB	6
Semiramis	$25,000	2	Rent	Massage, doula	P/EB	6
Skylar	$60,000	4	Rent	Stay-at-home mother	None	3
Theia	$20,000	4	Rent	Midwifery student	Public	4
Venus	$150,000	4	Own	Therapist	P/EB	6
Veronica	$45,000	4	Own	Midwife	P/EB	6

Note 1: * This participant declined to state a figure but reported medium to a high range of income.

Note 2: The abbreviations and codes that I've used in this analysis:

[a] Insurance:	P/EB	Private/Employer-based
[b] Education:	1	Elementary school (K–6th)
	2	Middle school (7–8th)
	3	High school / GED (9th–12th)
	4	Some college/Trade school (Associates, Trade certificate)
	5	College graduate (Bachelors)
	6	Post-college (Graduate school, Masters, Doctorate)

Emotional pleasure was the most common aspect of pleasure reported by my study participants, present in every interview (along with mental pleasure, as these were often interconnected). In some ways, emotional pleasure was the least complex in terms of my analysis.

Relationality was the most central factor in shaping emotional pleasure. Callie's first-and-only hospital birth (although difficult because of complications necessitating an induction) was a site of profound emotional pleasure for her. Callie, as a Black woman, a public health scholar with a strong orientation toward Black feminist praxis and a deep awareness of the challenges of birthing within the US sociocultural context of institutional and obstetric racism, had created a support team to protect her peace in the hospital. She had carefully chosen her obstetrician and her doula team, all Black and all in a warm relationship, which helped her feel connected and safe. She reflected: "...when I look back at pictures,

I look really tearful, but I didn't feel—like I didn't feel sad. I didn't feel overwhelmed. I felt really, like, whole and at peace."

For Romi, who is a White-passing Moroccan Jew, during her arduous first hospital birth experience, she experienced being seen, supported, and centered, which also resonates with this theme of relationality. During our interview, she shared:

> I felt seen in a way that I've never felt seen in my entire life before ... I think there's a part of me that just so wanted to be seen ... all of these people are here for me for my baby ... It's sort of like a little bit embarrassing to admit, right? It's like, "Oh, I love this attention." But I did. I loved this attention, right? And I loved, like, everything that came with it.

The *relational space* around the birthing person emerges as a foundation upon which emotional pleasure can manifest, and as particularly critical within institutional birth settings.

This was true in autonomous birth center settings as well. The relational space around Cande also impacted their birth as a non-binary queer Latine/x. In Cande's first-and-only birth in a birth center, emotional pleasure was linked to their mental state as "ecstatic joy" or "euphoric joy" and to their connection with their partner. As they put in during our interview:

> [I experienced] complete calm to like moments of just like ecstatic joy ... But also ... right after the birth when like, they gave me [the baby] to hold, because we were keeping the sex, like, a secret we didn't know. And so, we look, and we didn't have a name ... I was like, "Okay," and I just looked at my partner and there was just like these like emotions of like, euphoric joy. And also, like, clarity and like, and I was like, "Oh, this is the name." Like, I was like, half-crying. I was sort of red. I was definitely exhausted. But just full of life.

Relationality also made a meaningful difference in Malika's first-and-only hospital birth, which was, for the most part, a painful and arduous process. During a special moment, emotional pleasure and catharsis had suddenly overtaken her as her Reiki-trained ob/gyn guided her through a healing experience. During our interview, she described:

> I just—I like remember hearing like the voice—it was the sound of the woman's voice. I felt like it was just me and her only in the room. She did ask me questions about my childhood. And I did cry. Because I was—it was—I guess it was so so so touching or so personable or so tender

> still, that I had—that that was the emotion that came out. And I just remember the voice, and just feeling like, you know, it was—it was okay for me to go through what I was going through. I'm safe. I'm okay.

Malika's emotional pleasure was directly tied to her sense of connection with this practitioner, in the face of her real and present fear of mistreatment as a Black woman navigating birth, which for her had begun at a freestanding birth center with a subsequent hospital transfer due to complications (meconium).

Relationality was a salient theme in the home birth interviews as well. For Melissa, a mixed-race Black Latina woman, the emotional pleasure in her home birth was born of a sense of triumph over a previous hospital birth (that had involved a non-consensual episiotomy). She was eager to give voice to the pleasure of her second birth experience. In her words:

> I experienced pleasure more on an emotional and spiritual level. And I was excited to do this interview because I feel like I don't really ever hear about that part of labor. I was just—I just wanted to share my story.

Like Malika, emotional pleasure was tied to relationality in Melissa's account:

> I found myself having to give up control. And not only that, but like lean on my husband, my birth team in a way that I had never leaned on anyone before. Where I experienced all of my pleasure, really, it was, yeah, it was being in this heightened state of discomfort, but like, at the same time, being very aware that I was so loved and cared for. Um that it was, it was just trippy to me. Because it was my like, I guess really the first time experiencing that level of vulnerability, but like, mixed with everything else that was going on.
>
> I just loved my husband so much more. And we don't even like—he's very in tune with me and nature and the whole process. We didn't practice how he would support me, like he just knew what to do. And, and that was, I dunno I guess that was the enlightenment for me, or that, "Wow, this, this experience," although it was like screaming and long and it tested all of my physical abilities, it was still very loving. It was like it was that constant love at all times. And then you top it off with a baby. And that's like the epitome of love. It was nice.
>
> And another thing maybe compounded by the fact that I was home and my daughter was there. I was surrounded by people who I trusted. It was just like, love overflow. It sounds so cheesy, but it was just, like

> that, such a warm feeling. And then it was August, and it was hot and sunny. It was just perfect.

Melissa's account demonstrates the micro to macro levels almost spherically enwrapping and permeating her birthgiving in many layers of pleasure. In these ways, emotional and mental pleasure were often entwined, and were patterned by the *relational space* around them, even in the midst of pain. Next, I distinguish emotional from mental pleasures because this distinction offers a more refined understanding of the study participants' pleasurable birth experiences.

Mental Pleasure

Mental pleasure, also present in every interview, includes mental states that tend to go beyond or contextually ground emotional states. Some examples include a sense of safety, relaxation, or feeling in control (or not). Some mental pleasure experiences leaned toward intellectual ideation, knowing, positive evaluation, cognition, or the study participants' interpretation of space, time, and body. What I've called *mental pleasure* also tended to co-arise with emotionality in the interviews (such as "feeling confident" arising from a mental sense of "having control"). I also coded altered states of consciousness such as feeling "high," "euphoric," "zen," or "out of body" as mental pleasure. I came to refer to the participant's mental and emotional states as their birth *head space*. For some, their pleasurable mental states I also coded as *spiritual pleasure*, if described as such by the participant.

For some, the mental pleasure came with simply realizing that they were in labor. During our interview, Callisto, in her first-and-only home birth, shared just how glad she had been to be in labor at long last. In her words:

> I think the best part about the birth was giving birth, because not only was it just the most (LAUGHS) insane (LAUGHS) experience ... Um, but yeah, I had a lot of pregnancy symptoms. So, the most pleasurable part about all of it was just being able to hold my baby and know that I wasn't pregnant anymore.

Callisto's quotation above resonates with the cognitive framing I've used to define mental pleasure because her emotion was based on her intellectual assessment of what it meant that she was finally in labor (the anticipated end of her various unpleasant pregnancy symptoms).

In a different way, Nava spoke to mental pleasure in the sense of being in an altered state of consciousness during her first-and-only birth in an autonomous birth center. During our interview, Nava described the mental state that she experienced as follows:

> … just this like, intense high. I mean, I've done drugs before. And it wasn't at all like—You know? This was, like, the most real high I think I've ever—you know? Because it was completely natural. It was completely from within—within me, not something external. And it felt really right. And I would love to go back to that moment and re-experience it. Yeah, I guess I'll have my next births and they'll be different. But it was—yeah. Like, I feel close to that moment, but also far away because I haven't felt anything so intense, so beautiful—ever.

Similarly, Romi shared that the profound mental and spiritual pleasure (which I elaborate on below) that overtook her during her long and difficult first birth in a hospital had left her craving the experience of more births:

> I had been laboring; I was in a lot of pain. My doula was there. And I remember the lights were dim. And I kept on kind of passing out in between contractions because I was in so much pain, and I was mainly so exhausted. That's what I remember. I was just fatigued. And then I remember I have this image in my mind of kind of like lying back with my eyes closed with like a slight smile on my face, which is kind of bizarre, but I just remember that. And I remember feeling kind of like this wave of euphoria, almost like I was like, floating, like, this is where I'm supposed to be. It was sort of like, it was like, separate from time. It was sort of like an out of body experience. And the only way I can describe it is like being on drugs. You know, I'm not someone who does drugs, I'm very easily affected by chemicals. And so, but it was like this high. And I feel like since I've given birth, I've been chasing that high, literally, which sounds crazy, but whatever part of your brain is stimulated by, you know, by like, addiction, I feel like that part of my brain was stimulated.

These above descriptions suggest that a wide range of mental pleasure experiences are possible in birth. On one side, the study participants' typical states of mind included pleasurable cognition, interpretation of events, and sense of knowing. On the other side are altered states of consciousness that included "highs" described in a variety of ways, articulated as euphoria, bliss, beauty, being in a trance, out-of-body, dreamy, far away, in one's own world, being on drugs, floating, and the like. Some participants described these states with spiritual or religious language. Also, some participants connected these kinds of ethereal notions with biological explanations, such as a rush of oxytocin, endorphins, and generally "hormones." Some described these mental pleasure states as including physical sensations, which I cover next.

Physical Pleasure

In this section I introduce the term "physical pleasure" to refer specifically to the pleasurable bodily sensations experienced during birth, which I differentiate from "sexual pleasure" in the section to follow. All but two of my interview participants (21 of the 23) had reported physical pleasure as an aspect of their pleasurable birth experiences. Physical pleasure often involved the visceral sensations of birthing itself from having enjoyed the sensations of contractions, cervical or vaginal stretching, the intensity, effort, or physicality of the experience to feeling the movement and the eventual emergence of their newborn(s). Interview participants also described the physical sensations of affection, support, and comfort measures such as enjoying the sensation of water in a shower or birth tub, of being held, of movement, massage, or the relief of tension from counter-pressure in terms of physical pleasure. Participants had frequently distinguished between physical pleasure that had not been sexual from sexual pleasure, often rejecting a sexual framing for what might otherwise be socioculturally interpreted as a sexual experience based on where or how a given sensation had occurred within the birthing body, such as the reproductive organs.

Marion's home birth account conveys the many layers of pleasure experienced in concert. Here I pull just a couple of excerpts that demonstrate physical pleasure well. During our interview, Marion (a White cis straight woman about birthing vaginally for the first time) described:

> I could just feel her head right there and I could just feel it jiggling as I moved. And it felt really good. Just move my hips and just kind of feel that cervical opening. Like that felt really good! And I—it didn't feel super painful, and the contractions just demanded my attention. They weren't painful. They just demanded my attention.
>
> Physically, the feeling of dilation was so satisfying ... There was a pinching, so I guess you would call that a negative feeling but, um, it wasn't really—like I could just feel exactly where she was, and I could just almost like kind of roll her head around is what it felt like—just like rolling her head around on top of my cervix, and I would just kind of, like, roll my hips into that, and it felt pretty good. And—I was just so proud of myself that I was so focused! Because I guess I would describe my pain tolerance as very low. And I knew that it was—I knew that the

> squeezing was hurting, and I was aching, but it wasn't anything that made me want to get away. It was just like, "Hey, you're doing good!" Like I felt proud of myself. That was very positive.

Marion's account wove back and forth between her pleasurable physical sensations (cervical dilation feeling good), mental assessments (of doing good), and emotional layers (feeling proud). She also grappled with the language around pain itself, at points having contradicted herself; in my sense, it had been a confrontation of the limitations of language for such very intense, rich sensations.

In Sankofa's account of one of her three home births, physical pleasure emerged from within a mental state of safety and connection, as a physical transfer of what she called "energy." During our interview, she described:

> I just felt so safe to just be there and know that the midwife is in the other room so if anything happened, she's here. But that moment of us just like hanging on to each other, and I would sleep in between, and then I would feel a contraction, I would just kind of like, tighten my grip a little bit on him, and he would tighten his grip back on me. And I could feel like that energy kind of going back and forth between us. I would ride the wave and then like, go back to sleep. And that's how we did like the whole night ... it was incredibly powerful, but incredibly peaceful at the same time, if that makes sense. Whereas the contractions I never felt I got to the point in that labor I was like, "Oh my gosh, this is so painful." It felt really strong and really powerful! But it also felt really safe and peaceful.

Here, Sankofa (a Black cis heterosexual woman) had described an exchange of energy between her body and her husband's body and connected her physical pleasure with their relational space, a sacred container she and her husband created. The emotional and mental pleasure entwined with the physical in the deep connection, safety, and peace their bond provided during her birth.

Bree (a Vietnamese American heterosexual cis woman) gave birth to her first child at the age of 25 at home and pain-free, and, during our interview, had summarized her physical experience of pleasure as follows:

> So, for me, it was just very sensual. Like I could actually feel her moving in there. I could feel every contraction. I could feel the good and the bad. But for me, it wasn't—there was no pain involved. It was just a lot

> of pressure. And I don't even know how to describe it. It was like, I just felt passionately alive.

Again, it appears to me that the study participants had been grappling with the language of physical sensations, intensity, and differentiating the good and the "bad" in the birth context.

During our interview, Skylar (a White cis heterosexual woman) also described the sensations of the physical pleasure during her second birth in terms of pressure and release, something like a massage. In her words:

> I was having the contractions. Like, they didn't feel bad. They just were like—it was just extremely joyful and pleasurable. It wasn't like—I guess I really don't know how to describe it … But it just—it was, it was exciting because I'm sitting here having my son and I— there was just joy. It was easy. It was painless. It was all of the above. (LAUGHS) … I would say it was kind of like massage? Okay. Okay. Just kind of like, my body just kind of—it was just moving. And, like, it just—it felt like—I guess it kind of felt like there was just kind of a release. And that—kind of similar to how when you have a massage, like there's pressure and but then there's comfort in that pressure too. Kind of similar to it.

Hospital births also involved physical pleasure. Araceli had shared during our interview about her second hospital birth (having practiced hypnobirthing techniques in preparation), that her physical sensations had been those of embodied ecstasy:

> I was ecstatic. I don't know how else to describe it. I had all the hormones! It was amazing! It was super! I didn't mean that I had an orgasm because that's not true. But I was definitely in this, like, very embodied zone where it all felt perfect. And as I wanted it, and connected, and like super powerful.

Semiramis had experienced something similar during her first-and-only hospital birth. In her words:

> It's really hard to explain. It was sort of like a choir singing. (LAUGHS) You know, just like, like, just the most beautiful—if it was a sound, and I'm a little bit synesthetic, like, I've always kind of associated taste with sound or feeling a sound or like various, like, different senses. So, I mean, it was like a choir singing in my body.

She continued:

> I just, I totally pushed at my own pace. And it was—I didn't—no one told me when to push, and I felt really good to just—I was like (LAUGHS)—I just—it felt amazing. Like it was the best feeling to just like push when I needed to and just—and it was intense. It was a really intense, glorious drive to like—you know. And then I definitely felt pleasure in that, you know. And then when she was crowning, I felt what they call the "ring of fire," you know, just like this radiant, intense pleasure stretching opening like—it was beautiful. It was like this burning, amazing feeling and—and that is what got me through, you know, her coming out … And when I was done, like immediately, I was like, "Wow, I could do that again." Actually, I'd like to.

This longing for more births was shared by several interview participants, especially those who experienced emotional pleasure, altered states of consciousness (mental pleasure), and physical pleasure combined.

Cande's description of the physicality of their pleasure is rich, nuanced, and marked with metaphor. They mention pleasure in physical exertions and overcoming limitations, as well as an "energy force" to depict their experience as something volcanic:

> [Giving birth was] one of the biggest workouts I've ever had. And I'm pretty active. Like, during my pregnancy, I was working out almost every day. And I'm a big camper and hiker and played sports, like traditional sports growing up and everything … I don't know if you've ever exerted yourself to the point of almost collapsing. And in that sort of exertion, there's like the feelings of like, I keep going, keep going, keep going, keep going. And then you plateau, and you're sort of like "I've overcome it." So, there were definitely moments of that. And then, in the moment that he was like actually physically coming out, it was like I reached that pinnacle peak of like ... it wasn't exertion, but it was like this energy force. And it's kind of hard to explain because it was just like this whole energy was peaking. All peaking, right, as it came out. It sort of just shot—exploded … Maybe like a volcano, and if you could imagine the lava coming to the surface, and then as soon as it hits it sort of like spreads out everywhere and then sort of falls down. The moment of birth was probably right as it hits like that volcano opening. So, it was like this crazy burst of energy that then floated up. And then my head space through it, most of coming up to it was like focusing on meditating through and visualizing. And so, trying to not control what was happening because I couldn't, but just releasing

> and letting go. And I tend to like to control things. (LAUGHS) So that was really hard. But as he was coming down the birth canal, like I said, I could almost basically see him coming down, and I could feel him moving through the birth canal. And then, when he came out, there was the moment between him coming out and before I held him, there was this weird feeling of loss. Like something all of a sudden was gone. And so, it was like, as soon as they put him in my arms, I like had to really grab onto him to hold them because that was like the rejoining of what was lost. And that sort of, I think, was like joy, ecstatic, and everything sort of culminating in like that space of loss.

Most of the study participants who had described their physical birth sensations as pleasurable in their interviews did not convey those experiences in terms of sexuality. Romi, who'd had two hospital births, was quite clear about her rejection of sexual language for the profound pleasure she experienced:

> I don't like that term [orgasmic birth] because for some women, they experience orgasms during birth. It wasn't like that for me. And so, when I've told women about it, they're like, "Oh, did you have an orgasm?" I'm like, "No, it was not sexual at all." And even my doula recommended the film "The Orgasmic Birth," and I was like, "Yeah, but it wasn't orgasmic. Can we not sexualize it?" For me, personally.

Here, Romi highlighted tension in the ways physical birth sensations are interpreted as sexual or not, and pushback on any sexualized framing imposed on what had been experienced as distinctly non-sexual. Sensations in the reproductive body, for many participants, were not by definition *sexual* sensations. Perhaps for these participants, the pleasurable mental and emotional layers of their birth experiences had determined the interpretations of pleasurable sensation as having been sexual or not. In the absence of erotic desire, sexual arousal, or a particularly sexual style of relationality, physical sensations in the reproductive body (the uterus, clitoris, vagina, pelvis, and vulva) might not have been experienced as sexual, but rather as distinct and unique to birth. Next, I present sexual pleasure as experienced in the context of birth, as described by my study participants.

Sexual Pleasure

Sexual pleasure was held as quite distinct from physical pleasure for most of my interview participants. As such, in my analysis I have distinguished sexual pleasure from physical pleasure based on the presence or absence of sexual desire or the stirrings of the erotic. Eroticism and sexual desire typically started in the mind and then colored the physical sensations as sexual. Sexual pleasure had also started, for some participants, in the body and then brought the mind along for the ride. For some participants, sexual pleasure happened unexpectedly alongside other physical sensations. Others intentionally stimulated sexual pleasure with sexual interactions, intercourse, or self-touch. For sensations of the genitals or other sexually associated areas of the body, descriptions often included either an explicit emphasis or rejection of their sexuality. In these data, sexual pleasure is not synonymous with orgasmic or ecstatic states, although some participants mentioned "orgasm." Many of my participants had used the word "orgasm" (or related words) as a homolog or stand-in for something they found difficult to put into words. Generally, "orgasm" had not been embraced as an ideal reference point to convey their lived experience. To complicate this a bit further, during some interviews, the "orgasmic" label was rejected as a sexual one but rather was used as a kind of short-hand for a range of sensations in birth, and without eroticism. For this reason, I coded experiences as "sexual pleasure" in my data analyses only when the interview participant had explicitly labeled their own experience as having been sexual or erotic.

For Nava, sex was a part of her labor story, but just before her waters broke. She'd had sex with her husband before she'd realized that she'd been in labor with her first child:

> … we had sex, and immediately after, my water broke in the bed. And I wasn't sure, so I just noticed like a whole bunch of fluid, and I thought, "Okay, this could be something else; I want to make sure." So I went to the bathroom, and then more water started coming out, and it was clear. And I realized that okay, this is happening … And, and then immediately after I went to the bathroom, I started feeling really, really intense contractions. So right away, I'm—it's like, "Okay?" I wasn't expecting it to be so suddenly … I read about the different stages of labor, and I took a course, and I learned about the hormones and the stages and all that, and then this was kind of sudden.

This sexual experience had put her birth in motion quite precipitously. Her labor lasted just two hours from first contraction to birth. But, overall, she had not described the other pleasurable aspects of her birth in terms of sexuality—just this sexual experience with her husband.

Some participants strategically used sexual pleasure in labor as a resource or tool. Throughout her first-and-only home birth, Pearl had strategically used sex during labor to support her process. While Pearl's desire for sex during labor had been powerful and primal, it was driven by a practical desire to shift her embodied state. She had wanted to match the intensity of the contractions somehow, and to do something that would help her to sink down into her body and to let go more deeply, rather than a need to satisfy an erotic desire in itself. During our interview, she explained:

> ... the day before [delivery], the contractions were really intense. So, I wanted to have sex and like get into my body and also in just a different head space. And so, we did, and it was really profound. It felt very intense. It was erotic. But my mi—I think my body took over so much that it shut my mind off a little bit more ... And feeling those huge contractions and then orgasming felt like, just massive. It just felt like a very, very deep, carnal space to get to ... I think sex helped me shift how I related to the sensation, and like gave me an alternative, like information that my body could do to help kind of ease into it more.

She continued:

> [After sex] I did feel like I could sink into it. My body just felt like more like mushier or something or like, like, I could—almost as if, like, you're at a dance party or something, or like you're at a place with music, and for whatever reason, you feel awkward. There's like an awkwardness, but then something shifts, and you get into it? (CHUCKLES) You know what I mean? (CHUCKLES) ... I definitely think it was more of a physical space of pleasure, that—So I had to turn off my mind for my body to experience it. And then I feel like my body gave the feedback loop up to my brain to be like, "Hey, this is cool. This is good," you know? And so, I think it was more my body that, yeah, allowed that kind of like, went back up and told my brain like, "Hey, chill out, this is good." And then my, but my brain was trusting my body and saying, "Ah yeah, this is pretty cool."

Cande, also in labor with their first child, engaged in some intentional sexual self-stimulation during their labor: "I did orgasm during, like, during labor ... Like when I first started having contractions. I remember ... I actually, like, had orgasms while I was like—as a way to counteract the contractions ... which, I guess, is a huge thing about pleasure." Similarly, the study participants who had intentionally self-stimulated their own sexual pleasure (typically clitoral touch) during labor had only done so within the privacy of their own homes.

Others experienced sexual stimulation from therapeutic touch during their births. Veronica had, during our interview, reported a great deal of surprise at what she considered sexual pleasure as her midwife had applied oil to assist the vaginal opening in stretching as her baby had slowly begun to crown:

> There were these unexpected moments of, like, physical pleasure. Um, and at one point, the midwife, like, as my son was crowning—she was mostly very, very hands-off. But she started like—he must have been crowning up pretty good, 'cuz I mean, I didn't have any pain meds. So I remember all of this and like the burning, and that there was so much pressure and burning, but then, I don't know if she had, like, gel on her fingers or what she was doing, but she was like, running her fingers around the, like, introitus, like that [gestures her fingers swirling in a spiral], stretching vaginal tissue. And that felt actually really good, in a way where it, like, part of me was like, "Why is she doing that?" Like, "That's like ..."—it was like sexual pleasure. It was like, "That's not what I was expecting." You know, it was very momentary, and it was also, like, it was okay. You know, I didn't feel violated or anything, but an unexpected really good feeling in the midst of all of this other, like, hard to—hard-to-hold feelings.

In a similar way, Venus had also reported sexual stimulation from the pressure that her midwife applied to her clitoris, and how that had impacted her second home birth experience. In her words:

> … she put pressure on my clitoris a little bit, actually kind of a lot. Part of it she was trying to contain, but then also she was encouraging me to just feel pleasure … I was able to—you know, rock a lot and I could feel that embarrassment but also like kind of the pleasure … the sensation of the clitoral pressure and like the pleasure of that rocking motion and like just like ... I felt literally like that flower opening. It really, really, like-—helped. And my midwives weren't even there for ten minutes before the baby came out.

Venus had also practiced perineal massage to rehearse relaxing and releasing her pelvic floor. In combination with this preparation and the clitoral contact, Venus had been able to move into her physical experience rather than resist it, which she believed had made her experience of pleasure possible. She had also found the pushing phase to be the most pleasurable of any aspect of her labor:

> … the most pleasurable, honestly, was when it turns to the pushing stage. Like, I'm sure a lot of people say that. I think it was that for me, that was about such a radical shift in hormones, or what's happening with our system. So, I was really happy to not be medicated so that I could experience all of that. Because, like, the transition time, I was just really aware of the fear. You know, which I know is the rush of adrenaline to kind of prepare you to take care of your baby if the baby is born in nature, right? So having that knowledge, somehow, I was able to tell myself that. And, and during the pushing, that's usually when both times my midwife would kind of, like, just touch my clitoris a little bit, or just hold my hand there. And it provided like this warmth and pleasurable sensation. And then, of course, there's just the moving really helped. And the idea that I could do something, finally, like with pushing. It just felt so good … we did the perineal massage … so, I was able to have the body recall and relax … That somehow, when I was being stretched in the pushing, I was able to relax those muscles, which gave way to more pleasure, experience, and sensation.

The feeling of the baby descending through her vagina toward birth had been another sexual experience of pleasure that Venus had spoken about with great clarity:

> Oh, I loved feeling the baby move down. I mean, I did love that! (LAUGHS). It was trippy, you know? … You know, at first, I was like, "Oh, I don't think it's gonna fit!" My midwife is like, "Yes, he will." (LAUGHS). And so yeah, the pain stopped when I relaxed. Which I think is really hard to do, maybe. But I do think that practicing the perineum massage helped a lot. And having the midwife there who I was comfortable with, like, to know that it was okay if I rocked my hips while her hand was cupping my vulva. You know, that was—it's like a very intimate thing (LAUGHS) and vulnerable and weird … I remember just thinking "Wow, like, I bet a free birth—or if I was even more comfortable—could be like, a lot more easeful?" You know, if I had actually been able to pleasure myself more or surrender more into that.

Venus had also mentioned her intellectual alignment with the concept of "ecstatic birth," and had related this concept to her experience as follows: "I was very fascinated by this idea of ecstatic birth because I could really see how it [birth] opened me. You know? And, and the mixture of that intensity, it was almost hard to tell the difference between the pleasure and pain." Venus had resonated with the term "orgasmic birth" as well, as she explained:

> I would say it's orgasmic in that feeling of—there's all these waves of the contractions. And then with the release, it's kind of like the biggest orgasm ever. (LAUGHS) ... I don't think I've ever felt more embodied than when I was giving birth (LAUGHS). You know? Fully alert, fully there (LAUGHS).

Venus had intentionally engaged her sexuality and thus had given birth in an embodied way, with all of herself. It follows then that her experiences of birth pleasure spanned the full gamut from emotional and mental pleasure to spiritual, physical, and sexual pleasure, even while she had also experienced pain in various shades. She had oriented her head space and body space toward having pleasurable experiences, and the relational space around her, including her midwife, partner, and friends, had aligned with this orientation, within a context that supported her pleasure: her own home. Combined, the result was a rich tapestry of birth pleasure; experiences that she relished in recounting to me during our interview.

Aleks, in giving birth at home to their fourth child, had integrated sexuality into their birth experience, in some ways as a function of their identity as an agender lesbian. They had, during our interview, described this birth using relational language, naming interpersonal dynamics clearly at play in their home birth experience. They had also engaged their entire birth process from a place of unapologetic sexiness while drawing parallels to their erotic life and queer identity:

> I just allowed myself to be very primal, animalistic, and like, move with the labor instead of like worrying how I'm seen. But there was really something to having queer women and queer people around me. I had a queer friend come over as well, with whom like we have flirtatious friendships and, and there's also something to the doula being queer. Like, I was naked in front of these women. And there is a pleasure to that. And not only was I naked in front of these women, and we were all queer, but I was like, able to be just open, right, and like, peeing, and bleeding, and pooping. I had a bucket. (LAUGHS) I was l joking around with them. And then I was like bearing into the bucket, and all of these things were coming out, and every once in a while, my wife would empty it ... and I just thought, "What an incredible experience!" where it was like embodied and flirtatious and sexual, and they were joking about other things and like, just talking to each other, and I just was like, first of all, I find all of these people attractive simultaneously.

> Second of all, I'm in love with what's taking place right now, because it's taking some—labor takes time. It's a process ... I'm just, I just was thinking, you know, like, how much this feels like the sex parties that we attend, to some extent with people around, kind of moving around and doing their own thing, but you're also doing something with your body, but like, times a thousand, because like, there's a baby coming, like, you know? So, it was a very queer experience, very sexual in that way ... the way I was delivering was just unapologetic. It was, like, strong. And it was not the divine feminine. It was like, you know, the more contemporary version of, like, someone empowered.

Aleks had experienced this birth at the intersections of their gender and sexual identities and in defiance of many sociocultural normativities in terms of birth setting (at home), choice of queer support people (queer Black midwife and doula), and their life partnership (a bi-racial queer lesbian marriage). They had embarked on this home birth experience after having experienced two previous cesareans and one previous vaginal birth in an autonomous birth center. Some of my readers might think that the odds for a pleasurable birth experience had not been in their favor, given the various oppressions poised against them. However, as I further expand upon in Chapter 5 of this book, Aleks had been able to leverage their identities and relationships as potent resources in birth, thereby fostering and protecting their unique birth head and body spaces.

Debbie's birth experiences had been quite different in terms of sexual pleasure from the interviews that I have covered above. She had twice given birth in a hospital; her first birth was extremely traumatizing and abusive, and the second was much more positive. In both, she had experienced many complications and non-consensual interventions, but also both times, immediately after birth, Debbie had suddenly been overtaken with an all-consuming wave of lust. As she described:

> ... right after birth, for both of my children, this—what I thought was like this really unusual surge of lust overcame me, and like—within minutes after the birth. And then—and I was married to two different men, and it really was not a reflection on our lust for each other, or the fantasticness of our relationship. It was, it was totally different. It was purely physical ... Sexual, overwhelming lust. Yeah. Sexual drive ... It was a complete and utter overwhelm of my response. I couldn't fight it. I couldn't even think through it ... it lasted probably like 30 minutes, but my husband would have nothing to do with it. But I still felt it like, like, in my womb, in my, in my clitoris, in my breasts. I felt the tingling,

> the sensation of the sexual stimulation, and in my mouth. I just wanted to—I just wanted to deep kiss and go at it. Like, I like—I dunno. Like I never had … it was not an orgasm. It was—It was—it was that place before orgasm where you're like, "I gotta have this. I gotta—don't stop. I want this. I want this. I want this." It was before that. And I imagine if—if, we were in another time and place with another mindset, it could have been pretty fun.

In summary, fewer study participants experienced sexual pleasure and their experiences varied greatly. Sexual pleasure entwined with the birthing person's identity, the birth context, and the sexual interpersonal experiences of birth care. Sexual stimulation had been intentionally generated or had spontaneously arisen. For some participants, sexual pleasure had involved self-stimulation, for others, sexual intercourse. For others, sexual pleasure had taken them completely by surprise. Sexual pleasure had also occurred at different times during the birth process: during contractions, pushing, or immediately postpartum. The emotionality of these sexually pleasurable birth experiences spanned a broad spectrum of emotions, including embarrassment, awkwardness, unapologetic sexual exuberance, and overwhelming lust. Overall, sexual pleasure was the least common and most varied form of birth pleasure in this typology.

Spiritual Pleasure

Some participants' descriptions of pleasure had invoked spiritual language and spiritual interpretation. When these types of descriptions emerged during interviews, they brought yet another layer of experience to the participants' emotional, mental, physical, or sexual sensations. Spiritual language also conveyed how the participants contextualized these sensations. Spiritual framing provided frameworks for the interpretation of birth pleasure: it shaped how they had given their birth experiences meaning. I did not attribute spiritual themes unless the study participant directly named their birthing experience as having been spiritual in nature, which largely tied to their spiritual identities (for a summary of the study participants' spiritual and religious identities, see Table 2.5).

As Table 2.5 clearly shows, most of the study participants identified as "spiritual but not religious." Of those who identified with an organized religion, four were Protestant Christians, one was Catholic, and two were Jewish. Two participants identified as pagan or polytheistic, one other as an atheist witch, one secular humanist, and one as interfaith. One participant

TABLE 2.5 The Study Participant's Demographics: Spirituality and Religion

Pseudonym	*Spirituality and Religious Identity*
Aleks	Pagan Atheist Witch
Araceli	Raised Catholic, now SbnR[a]
Bree	SbnR
Callie	SbnR
Callisto	SbnR
Cande	Raised Catholic, now SbnR
Chandra	Catholic
Dalisay	SbnR
Debbie	Pagan
Fabia	SbnR
Malika	Christian (non-denominational)
Marion	Christian (non-denominational)
Melissa	SbnR
Nava	Jewish, Observant
Pearl	SbnR
Raquel	No religious beliefs
Romi	Jewish, Conservative Sephardic
Sankofa	SbnR
Semiramis	Polytheistic
Skylar	Christian (non-denominational)
Theia	Christian (Lutheran)
Venus	Interfaith
Veronica	Secular Humanist

Note: [a] SbnR: Spiritual but not religious

reported holding no religious beliefs. Comparing these different identity groups to each other revealed no significant patterns—every loose category in spiritual identity had widely varied in how salient their spiritual or religious identity had been during their birth. The most salient pattern was that those participants with the most rigorous spiritual or religious practices were more likely to describe the pleasure that they'd experienced during birth with spiritual or religious language, and thus, I have coded their pleasure as "spiritual pleasure." Participants who experienced spiritual pleasure in birth spanned all spiritual/religious categories and sociocultural positions. During our interviews, some participants shared more than others about how they'd had the opportunity to engage their religious and cultural identities in their birth processes. These had taken the forms of meditation, prayer, and embodied visioning. For example, during Skylar's home birth, she had reached nine centimeters of cervical dilation when her labor had suddenly stalled. She shared about her use of prayer in those moments:

> We sat and we waited until noon … I just kind of walked out of the room for a little bit, went into the bathroom to have some time to myself, and I prayed. I was like, "I really want this to get done and finished, and I don't want her to think something is wrong, because things aren't moving anymore." And little did I know, at the time—I found out probably about a month later, my husband did the same thing, right when I walked away … And so I walked back in the room. Ten minutes later, it hit noon, and everything started up again. Strong. I could feel it. Like I could no longer talk through the contractions. But there was still no pain.

In this way, Skylar used prayer as a tool for releasing mental tension or worry, and perhaps this aided her labor process. Others used meditation or other spiritual practices. As I've previously noted and to recap here, Callie, for example, used meditation throughout her labor during her hospital birth:

> I had my whole team of folks like massaging my hands, massaging my temples. I was doing really good. Like, breathing—meditation really works. And I began to feel what I described as Zen-like. Folks around me were saying I looked like—I was doing the butterfly pose, I was sitting up with my legs bent in the butterfly stance, and I felt—and when I see pictures—I look really Zen. And I wasn't stressed. I was ready. Is like, the main way I can describe it. I was just focusing on my breathing.

Callie had also created a special ritual before she had begun to push, and the vision board she'd made with her husband was available and within sight throughout this phase of her birth:

> I actually asked everyone, meaning my husband, my mom, the doulas to leave the room because I had a special ritual to do with my daughter. And I did that ritual and had those emotions and then I called them back in the room. And I pushed for 30 minutes, and she came out. [laughs].

Again, here is an account of emotional release through spiritual practices, in this case a meaningful ritual and a spiritual anchor in the form of a vision board, that had supported Callie through her challenging birth process. In a different way, Sankofa had, during our interview, directly related spiritual understandings, specifically the concept of "chakras," to the embodied experience of giving birth:

> For me, the power in the root chakra is like so strong and building up. And then, when you actually feel like that urge to push, it's almost like you can feel all the chakras being like aligned, like right away, like, it's like quick, fast. Whereas normally you would have to sit and meditate for a long time to kind of bring all that energy up. It's like, instant. Like it's flowing through your body so quickly. And I think for me, because I only—I will never push like two or three times. It happens so fast, that feels so incredibly powerful and gratifying. That I almost wish like I could push a little bit longer [laughs]. Because to feel that feeling for so long. But you know, it happens so fast, and the strength of it. I'm like I always attribute to red raspberry leaf tea, but I'm like, "No, it has to be the chakras," you know, "working with you as well." I think. Cuz I've had people drink red raspberry leaf tea for like, you know, the second and third trimester and push for a long time. So, it has to be, you know, something else that's actually happening on a spiritual level kind of in your body. Obviously, baby's still there.

In this way, Sankofa (and others) interpreted their bodily experiences through her spiritual understandings, thereby engaging in their birth process as a whole being, including their Spirit. Other participants had not engaged their religious or cultural identities during the birth process itself but processed their birth experiences through relevant spiritual lenses postpartum (for example, Romi's birth, which I have fully described above). In sum, spiritual identity thematically arose during interviews as a source of comfort measures in birth, and spiritual pleasure was unlocked when those comfort measures were highly relevant, resonant, and powerful for the birthing person. Spiritual pleasure contributed to what I've called the birth head space (to peace of mind, to safety, autonomy, and joy in the space of birth). For this reason, most of the spiritual pleasure my participants described had involved what I'd coded within "mental pleasure" as "altered states of consciousness," although these altered states were experienced as spiritual in nature and were cast in spiritual language during the interviews. Next, I present some of those descriptions.

Veronica, as a midwife herself, had conceptualized her births as spiritual events, and shares this conceptualization with her patients:

> It is [spiritual]! I mean, sometimes, like, I tell my patients ... birth is this really amazing, like, physical, also spiritual and emotional event.

> And, you know, you are literally the portal through which this new being is entering the universe ... And, and, like, inside our bodies, that's where something comes from nothing ... I remember like, looking at my son ... when he was newborn, and just thinking, "Whoa," ... in my, like, endorphin high, I was like "Ten months ago no molecule of your body was ... where it is now." Like, you were a banana and a salmon swimming in the ocean and, you know, a beet growing underground, and a piece of wheat, you know, like, out on the plains wherever wheat grows." You know? And just being really kind of blown away that, like, ten months ago, this person wasn't here. And now here he is. You know?

She continued:

> I think that ... there's divine pleasure in creation and in being—being part of the universe coming into being. Like, what better thing is there than—than that knowledge that you are this little, tiny part of this cosmic unfolding? Like, I mean, that's—that's pleasure!

During our interview, Romi described the spiritual pleasure of her birth experience as follows:

> ... it was almost like a spiritual and religious experience, like accessing this other part of the human experience, like the, like the female experience, and which is obviously tremendously powerful and sort of like connects you to your history and all the women in the world. And it's just, it's powerful. I'm like, I'm getting emotional as I talk about it.

For Semiramis, "it also felt kind of like otherworldly, like spiritual or something. Like, I was expanding. But like, not just physically—there was just, like, this openness and freedom." This sense of expansiveness was one of the most cited aspects of spiritual pleasure. Another aspect of spiritual pleasure that three of my study participants shared, some rather hesitantly, was their having had a "vision." Veronica experienced what she had called a "vision," which she described as follows:

> ... I think because I had all these endorphins, like when I was pushing with him, I just remember having this like vision of the entire like spiral galaxy being compressed into the space of my pelvis as he was passing through it. And it was like very cosmic and, you know—I felt like I had touched God. You know? There was just this really profound experience

of feeling like I was one with the universe and like part of this, like, bringing creation into being and, you know? I mean, so that was, that was a whole other kind of pleasure.

During Venus's first birth, she had also experienced being with God in something of a vision:

> ... [birth was] one of the most profound spiritual experiences of my life ... I felt like I was a gateway. You know, almost like, with God, like asking me, you know, "Are you ready?" And I feel like I was shown, you know, in the same way that maybe a hallucinogenic journey or medicine journey, you know? I really felt when I moved into transition, that I was—you know, almost like, tested. Like I just remember feeling like God was showing me, you know, "This is life, this is responsibility, and are you ready?" And I got that, that the intensity of the experience of birth, that was part of the initiation. You know? And so, it was—it was—it was incredible!

After the birth of her second child, Venus had seen her friends as "glowing" and as "angels." During our interview, she described the experience:

> It's like this euphoric power. Yeah, like, I felt like the goddess herself. You know, it was—I didn't have as much as that dreamy, like spiritual connection as I did in the first time—it was really I felt like I was in between worlds. This was faster. But the strength and power were like, you know, amazing. And the euphoria was there because it was like I was on ecstasy. You know? Everything was so beautiful. Like, when my friends walked in, they literally looked like angels. You know? I felt like I saw them glowing and—(LAUGHS). I was really awake ... It was literally like feeling like I was on ecstasy. It was that euphoric.

Dalisay had also experienced a powerful vision that had deeply impacted her, a vision of her long-passed father as having been both present at the birth of her son and as having been one with it, as if reincarnated. Her account:

> I remember this was like this, this outer body experience that I had. And I remember saying it and I don't know why I said it. But I said "Oh, there's my dad," because I just saw my Dad's face. Like, if this baby was my dad, like—it was really bizarre. But my father has a picture when he was about four years old, that I remember. My dad passed away by the

> way, many years ago. He died when I was about 12. And so, I had my first baby at 31. So, you know, but a lot of years have passed ... And so, when I looked at this baby after birth, that four-year-old picture of my dad was what I saw as my baby's face, and I said, "That's my dad." Which was very bizarre because I remember saying it. And that's what I felt. Like I'm connecting with my father. You know? ... somehow, I felt like he was an incarnation of my father. Like that, that was it. Like this, this can't be anyone else, but my father kind of going back— returning to life, you know?
>
> ... the ability to be able to connect to my father was very special. You know? I haven't had that. Right. You know, he's been absent in my life physically for years and years and years. And so, spiritually, maybe we did connect somehow ... in some kind of an alternate reality. So, I think that's—to me, that's—that's the beauty of that.
>
> And it was—it was good to—and even if it's—I mean, I know maybe this whole reincarnation thing is not valid, or there's no—no—you know, it's not reality based—but—but—if it's—you know, it's like not having a father—(TEARS). He missed weddings, and all of these things—(CRYING)—(SIGH)—that was the one instance where somehow, he—you know—validates that, you know, he's still around. (SNIFFS). That he was there during childbirth. That somehow, he knows that this is his first grandchild with me. That was a blessing. It was a huge blessing for me (CRYING).

Here, spiritual pleasure, within a reconnection to a loved one, to her source of life, and to her lineage, had all emerged during the birth of Dalisay's first child. While she had struggled to fully integrate this vision, recalibrating her birth experience to a pleasurable interpretation had helped her to gain some clarity around what this vision had offered to her: an avenue for reconnection that she had accessed within this special birth realm, or head space, that she had found. Spiritual pleasure had enduring and profound effects on those study participants who had described their experiences as such.

To conclude, the birth process is experientially expansive. Each birth is unique, its very own heroine's and hero's journey. Many study participants left their ordinary selves to go on this quest, to cross the gauntlet of birth, face the peril and the pleasure, and through that journey grew as people to reach the other side. The experiences of birth pleasure that I have distinguished and described above are experienced within wholeness, perhaps layered, interrelated, or maybe within one large, fluid, experiential realm, a realm born from the internal, material, and relational conditions of their lives.

3

PAIN-FREE BIRTH

Pleasure and pain tend to be understood and experienced as opposites, although not always. In this chapter, I address my participants' experiences of pain-free birth, which some held as core to their pleasurable experiences of birth. These pain-free births fit into three categories: (1) pain-free without anesthesia (in whole); (2) partially pain-free without anesthesia; and (3) pain-free while partially anesthetized. Table 3.1 provides an overview of these pain-free birthing experiences. Seven of the 23 study participants reported pain-free experiences without the use of any type of pain medications or treatments (analgesia or anesthesia). Four more experienced aspects of their birth process as pain-free, also without analgesia. One additional birth involved epidural analgesia placed at the very end of labor (close to transition, around 10 cm dilation), so the labor experience up to that point was without pain medication. While their births were perhaps intense or at times uncomfortable, these 12 interview participants emphasized that birth, as a whole or in part, is not necessarily painful.

There are many layers of biomedical, pain-centric normativity baked into the language of birth in the United States. For participants who birthed pain-free, language played a critical role. These participants were more likely to invest attention and attunement to the sensory experiences produced by their own use of language, and to adjust their language choices in ways that were both intentional and strategic. As I describe below, several participants described their sensations as requiring their full attention or as entirely consuming but were careful to distinguish this intensity from pain. Many of the respondents aligned their language (with

DOI: 10.4324/9781003499428-4

TABLE 3.1 Birth Pleasure-Pain Spectra: Overview of Interview Participants Experiences

Pseudonym	*Birth Pleasure-Pain Spectra*						
	Birth Pleasure Typology					*Pain-free Birth*[a]	
	Emotional	*Mental*	*Physical*	*Sexual*	*Spiritual*	*Whole*	*In part*
Aleks	1	1	1	1			1
Araceli	1	1	1		1	1	
Bree	1	1	1			1	
Callie	1	1	1		1		
Callisto	1	1	1				1
Cande	1	1	1	1			1
Chandra	1	1	1			1	
Dalisay	1	1	1		1		
Debbie	1	1	1	1			
Fabia	1	1	1			1	
Malika	1	1					
Marion	1	1	1	1			1
Melissa	1	1			1		
Nava	1	1	1	1	1	1	
Pearl	1	1	1	1			
Raquel	1	1	1				1[b]
Romi	1	1	1		1		
Sankofa	1	1	1		1		
Semiramis	1	1	1		1		
Skylar	1	1	1		1	1	
Theia	1	1	1			1	
Venus	1	1	1	1	1		
Veronica	1	1	1	1	1		
Total[c]	23	23	21	8	11	7	5
Percent	100%	100%	91%	35%	48%	30%	22%

Notes:

[a] Pain-free physiological birth without analgesia

[b] Reported pain-free experience without analgesia for most of labor, increased pain with Pitocin administration, and received an epidural due to concerns over fetal heart tones. Shortly thereafter, she was found to be complete (10 cm) and instructed to push.

[c] This table summarizes the number of interview participants who reported ever having experienced the types of birth pleasure or pain-free birth that I have delineated in The Birth Pleasure-Pain Spectra (not the number of such pleasurable birth experiences, which might be more than one for the same birthing person).

varied degrees of consistency) with their desired mental or physical birth states and avoided words that triggered any tension, fear, or worry. This, they said, was a major aspect of how they evaded mental, emotional, and physical states that they did not want. For example, terms such as "surges" or "waves" of "energy" replaced "contractions." Cervical "ripening," "softening," and "opening" replaced the more clinical terms "effacement" and "dilation." Similarly, "transformation" was used in place of "transition" (the point in labor often considered the most painful, when contractions are the most frequent and intense as the cervix approaches full dilation). Some declined to use terms such as the "Ring of Fire," a term popularly used to describe the stretching sensation of the pelvic outlet as the baby's head emerges (crowning). This "ring of fire" language also renders normative and centers head-first crown-presenting deliveries (which not everyone has). First, I discuss births that were pain-free in full, then in part. Lastly, I discuss Raquel's first-and-only birth, which I call "pain-free partially medicated," because her labor (an induction) was largely pain-free and without pain medication until an epidural was placed just before she reached full dilation. For reference, I provide a summary of the participants' demographics and a snapshot of their birth contexts and experiences in the Appendix to this book.

Pain-Free Birth without Pain Medication

Chandra's interview conveyed a vivid story of a pain-free first birth experience (with twins, and without analgesia) in the hospital. At the same time, it is a saga in self-efficacy. Overall, her story is one of serene happiness and calm and yet is punctuated with interference by the oppressive sociocultural structures and violations of her consent that she confronted in the hospital as a young Black mother birthing twins in 1978. In subsequent chapters, I go into great depth about Chandra's experiences in terms of race and racism, class, relationship status, and privilege. Here, I focus only on the ways in which her birth was pain-free, in spite of those dynamics. At 19 years of age, she awoke one morning to hazily discover that her water had broken. In her words:

> My twins were 10 days past their due date. And the labor itself was wonderful. I mean, the only thing, you know—the having to go to the hospital part ... like, seven, eight o'clock [am], I felt something weird, and felt kind of, tossing and turning in bed a little bit. And then went back to sleep. And then, you know, approximately like nine-ish, I felt water. And I sat up and—I sat up and I was like, dazed and confused. But not, you know, not afraid or anything, but just kind of like high and silly ... I felt really warm. And I felt really high. And I felt good. ... I was like "I just love this place. I'm just so good." I just felt so good. I didn't feel any pain.

The only times that Chandra reported being out of her high, comfy, dreamy head space or in any state of discomfort were when other people interfered with her peace. This happened at a few points during her first birth. The first time was when she called her mother to let her know that she was in labor, and her mother's response was that of surprise and fear, and that got Chandra upset and afraid momentarily. She described it in this way: "So once I got off, you know, my mother's trauma and—bless her soul—and I got to my friend's car, I kinda got back settled back into feeling dreamy and happy again." This part of her story can teach my readers, birthing people, and birth practitioners about the impacts of other people's projected birth traumas and negative past experiences, which can derail what might otherwise be a lovely birth experience. Shielding themselves from these negative sorts of influences is a major strategy that many of these participants used and is a theme in these pain-free birth stories, as I fully demonstrate below. Chandra stated:

> I didn't feel any pain. It didn't really feel like it was—"Was I contracting? I dunno? Yeah?" I wasn't tripping about it. But it was just like curious. It was just like, "This is interesting." "I'm leaking?" I felt serene … I felt joy. I really was happy. In my soul, in my cells, in my heart. I just felt so peaceful. It was a beautiful morning, October morning … I was, I was very relaxed. And I was very calm. And I was very happy. And I felt surges and surges and surges of—Oh my God, it just felt really good. (LONG PAUSE). People don't understand. (LAUGHS) You know? I just felt so good, like incredible well-being, incredible well-being. And that was a little afrai—a little afraid. But the fear was background, peripheral static. It was very—it was there. But it wasn't the major thing. The major thing was that I just wanted to find some way—I really wanted to find some way to find a cave and be by myself. I really didn't want to talk to people. I really just wanted my husband with me. And you know, and people were talking at me and there was other extraneous input that I did not want to deal with.

There was one specific moment during Chandra's first birth that she named as painful: when she'd had to defend her boundaries in the face of unyielding hospital staff who were keeping her husband from her and attempting to force her to accept interventions she did not want (specifically pubic shaving, a practice that has since fallen out of favor in the United States). In that moment, Chandra got angry and for the first time during her labor, she felt pain. In her words:

> I yelled. I looked this woman in the eye and yelled at her and sat up and crossed my legs. And the stripe of pain went across my belly. Because all

> the muscles were tightened up. I'm so sure. And then I felt so sad. And I was crying because I had been feeling so good. And I was wondering if that affected my babies. And if they were okay, now, you know because nothing was hurting. And why should it start hurting?

I highlight this moment of pain because it reveals important themes about The Pleasure-Pain Spectra and about pain-free birth, informed by Chandra's pain-free experience, which was deeply connected to her head space and emotional state. Disruptions to that state caused pain. An incident occurred that was a blatant act of obstetric violence. A nurse clandestinely administered a sedative to Chandra's intravenous solution and put her under not long after she had delivered her twins, without her informed consent. As a result, Chandra was rendered unconscious for much of the first day of her postpartum period. I go into greater detail about the obstetric racism and violence that Chandra experienced during this birth in Chapter 6 because it's just such powerful testimony. But in terms of her pain-free birth experiences, I want to also highlight her second birth.

Chandra came prepared and made sure that she would be shielded from any undue distress, or, as she put it, "any miscellaneous crazy nurses" during her second birth. As such, she was better protected, and as a result had an entirely pain-free birth experience, which she described in this way:

> I was just feeling, again very, very oxytociny, and very high and, and happy and pleasant, and I ate this wonderful meal with my kids. She [a neighbor] had made lasagna and salad, it was delicious homemade lasagna and salad. And a great big glass of milk. Delicious. And all my kids were fed and happy and playing and watching TV … with my neighbor's kids, and I was just feeling more and more dreamy and out of it. And again, I didn't feel any pain. Again, I just felt incredible well-being and happiness.
>
> I kind of sort of felt the urge to push, this feeling like I wanted to push, and again you know, it's challenging with my labors because I didn't feel any great, big, intense anything. Again, I would want to find a nice comfortable place and curl up and just wake up with the baby between my legs. I think that if I was left my own devices that would be what my body would totally have done.

Next, she summarized this entire birth so beautifully that it was hard for me to cut it down. While she was in early labor, her partner had brought her to the wrong entrance of the hospital, and so they found themselves walking a long way to the labor and delivery area. In her words:

> ... These long corridors in this hospital and then connecting corridors between buildings. We're just walking and walking and walking. And finally, I just sit down on one of these connecting corridors, like—it's glass connecting corridors between two buildings. I just sit down on the ground. I said, "I'm not moving because I really just need to have my baby." And it was very sunny again—funny—where I'd sat down was really sunny. And there was like this steel and glass, and it was warm. I just sat there. And he's like, "You gotta get up! You gotta get up!" And I'm like "No, I don't. I'm not going to. I'm fine right here. I'm fine. Right here." And he goes running off. And he finds an orderly with a wheelchair. And they scoop me up and put me in the wheelchair and they wheel me down the hall. Get me into L&D, they get me into the delivery room. And I'm complete. And they're like "Well, you can begin pushing whenever you'd like." And again, I think, I don't even think it was half an hour worth of pushing. And Joseph was one ounce away from being a 10 pounder ... But he was splendid, beautiful, shocking black hair. And just a gorgeous baby. So happy. Is it a bit—He smiled when he came, he was born, he smiled. They finally—"Oh look at him smiling!" Cuz people are still not used to—they were not used to unmedicated babies who can smile as soon as they're born because they're not loopy from drugs. So again, beautiful. I felt safe. I didn't have a stupid—I had educated my ex to watch out for any miscellaneous crazy nurses. So, with [my baby], I got to be skin-to-skin right away—put on him on me right away, and us breastfeeding within 15 minutes of his birth. And I just got to hold him and love him, like right away, and it was an excruciatingly beautiful experience.

Fabia had a similar head space of beauty, calm, and serenity during her second birth, which was unlike her first. She did not report her first unassisted home birth as pleasurable or pain-free, which she attributes to her fear. But her second birth was a very different experience, and that is the experience that she focused on most during our interview. She described a beautiful, simple day of pleasures, enjoying the wonderful sensations of her contractions as she moved through her day. That evening, labor intensified, and the contractions remained largely pain-free and "amazing." She reported mostly mental and emotional pleasure, but also physical pleasure. She had a calm, peaceful birth in her bathtub (which she did not really want to stay in, but the baby was coming too quickly for her to have time to get out of it). She then stayed in the tub for a good while after the birth. She reports the delivery itself as being somewhat painful but does not emphasize that pain. Her main experiential memories from this birth (her second) were a sense of surrender and calm confidence. She felt "fearless" and "serene," dwelling in the wonder of her new baby. In her words:

> I remember the first one because I guess because it was the first. It was—I was scared. As—even when I was a midwife in both. It was just what—what it happens when you don't know, when it's the first time you're there. But the second one I already knew. And I felt much more in control. I remember the contractions were not painful. I thought I was not in labor, because they were—I was so relaxed that the moment they started to become uncomfortable that they went down again … I would just close my eyes. And whenever I had a contraction—and—I remember that was just a wonderful feeling.

Her contractions were for the most part pain-free, except for one moment when her husband briefly left her birthing room. A flash of fear and grasping took hold. In her words:

> I had pain, I can remember that. I remember, there was—my husband was with me all the time. But he went to do something. And in that one contraction, he—I mean, I reached out and he was not there. I could feel that "No, no, no, no" this—and then he quickly came out. That was okay, then.

Delivery was also pain-free for Fabia, as here she described the tenderness that she brought to the process of crowning and delivery:

> I remember the moment when her head was out. And I was waiting for the rest of the body to come out. I remember, like, caressing her hair. And just feeling that moment like "This is it, in the next while she's going to be here." … I remember that moment between the head being out and the rest of the body coming out as just so amazing. Just like, trying to retain that moment forever is like, "Yep, this is it!" In the next contraction, she's going to be in my arms." And then she didn't make a noise, move anything for a while, a couple of minutes, three minutes, she was just so relaxed. I think she didn't realize she had been born, and she was just like, doing the same thing she was doing before … I remember when she opened her eyes, and I was just like, saying, "Hello, Mommy's here. Welcome." I remember that moment … She was just—like she was with her hands like this—next to her face, and

> just nice and calm. And then a little while after she opened her eyes, and she looked at me and it was just such an amazing moment. It's—it makes me realize how—how much birth is intervened and how very few births I've seen that are not intervened … all the memories I get is still of love, of wonderfulness, of "Wow, what is happening to me right now? This is just like the most amazing feeling!"

Bree also shared her amazement at the sensations of her labor, giving birth for the first time at home at the age of 25, with a committed intention to experience a pain-free "natural birth." She had rigorously prepared for this experience using hypnobirthing techniques. In her own words:

> I actually trained for months, like three months of listening to hypnotherapy and hypno-sessions, working on that to rewire the pathways of my thinking, in order to create this, you know, ideal experience. But I wasn't attached to the outcome, if that makes sense. It was, hey—like, anytime I had a fearful thought pop up like about birth, "Oh, it's going to be painful, it's going to be this is going to happen, blah, blah, blah," I would have to stop myself, you know, and rewire that pathway and tell myself "No," like, "birth is pleasurable—I'm not going to feel pain. I'm going to feel pressure instead. Just pressure. It's not pain. It's pressure." And that's exactly what I felt. You know, you—you bring your thoughts to reality. So, for me, it was just a wonderful experience that I was able to actually do what I set out to do.

Bree had the pain-free, pleasurable birth experience that she set out to achieve, and her experience of this process had been life-changing for her. In her words:

> I can't even tell you how amazing it was to be able to feel everything … for me, it was just very sensual. Like, I could actually feel her moving in there. I could feel every contraction. I could feel the good and the bad. But for me, it wasn't—there was no pain involved. It was just a lot of pressure. And I don't even know how to describe it. It was like, I just felt passionately alive … I really just had to surrender to the storm of sensations and let that current take me back home to her. It was incredible … I felt like I was high on drugs (LAUGHS). Like a lot of endorphins, probably. But I was just so completely blessed by this new life that I brought in, it was such an amazing experience. For me, it was just, it just felt like I had given birth to myself too. Because there's a lot of, you know, not fear, but I guess in a sense fear because I don't know what it's like to have a baby. So, it's just a fear of going into

> the unknown. But once you cross that bridge, you're the only person that can get through that. Nobody can hold your hand through it. You know, obviously, you know, your partner or husband can physically hold your hand, but nobody can actually walk you through the entire process of giving birth. You have to really dig deep and do that yourself. You can have support from external sources. But really, it's—it's an internal thing that you have to do.

Skylar also pursued a pain-free birth and ultimately experienced it during her second birth (first out-of-hospital), at home also at age 24. In a coming section, I spend more time on Skylar's birth story because she also experienced a tremendous amount of healing from the trauma that she had endured during her previous birth, so the excerpts that I share here are those that focus specifically on the pain-free birth experience that she had. But she would not have had that experience had she not known that it is possible and applied herself to its pursuit. In her words:

> With my first, I had learned about the possibility of having birth without pain. It was a totally new thought—idea, to me, and it—it kind of just, like rocked my mind a little bit. And I was like, "This is interesting," you know, "Okay, maybe, we'll see." And I kind of dug into it a little bit. Um, and I believed that I was going to have my daughter without pain. Um, but then induction day happened. A whole bunch of crazy stuff like that happened. And it didn't really work out for me. And then when it came—so I just, I used that time, though, from the time that she was growing to before I became pregnant with my second to just kind of study "Why—how could it even be possible?" And I was like, "Okay, you know what? This is something that I want." And so, I went after it. I started studying everything even deeper about why—how it was possible. And so, then after I had my pain-free birth with my son, I was like, "Okay, I need to share this, I need to let other moms know that this is possible. It's something that they can have if they want it."

For Skylar, her faith was one aspect that informed her path toward a pain-free birth experience—in pushing back against or shutting out the standard Judeo-Christian sociocultural narratives that she'd been familiar with in terms of birth being God's painful punishment for Eve's original sin. In her words:

> When I started studying about how pain-free birth is possible, I—faith is something huge for me. And so, when I started studying, like in the Bible about how—I know a lot of people think that God said it had to

> be painful and that was just kinda the end of the story. And so, I studied it—and how it didn't have to be. And that's really controversial for a lot of people. And I'm like, "That's okay." You know? Um, I knew outside of the Bible that it [birth] could be pain-free, and I knew with it [the Bible], it [birth] could be pain-free. And other people's opinions didn't matter to me, but I was gonna share it. Um, so when I got pregnant with [my baby], I just took that time and I dove into it. I said, "This is what is gonna happen, I'm gonna make it work." And so, I learned everything from how the muscles in the body work when you're having contractions. Why they don't have to hurt.

When her labor finally started, Skylar was thrilled that there was no pain, just pressure and tightness. She had no "ring-of-fire" or pain at delivery either. In her words:

> It was kind of like—It was like this pressure. And it was kind of like; I don't know how to describe it. But maybe like, if you could imagine like—okay, it's just kind of kind of sounds gross. But like when you're having to go to the bathroom. And you're just, you're like, kind of pushing a little bit. And then there's like tightness, your breath, like, your lungs. Like, they kind of go "Huhhhh," and you're like "huhhh." And so like, it was just like it was just this pressure and tightness that it made it so like my lungs wouldn't want, like I didn't want to breathe ... Um, but at the same time, like it didn't hurt, it was just pressure and tight. It just felt like an extremely powerful Braxton-Hicks. Um, and then um at about 12:30, I started feeling the urge to push. Um, and then at 12:40, my water broke. And the only part that I had any discomfort in this entire birth was when I had to get some constipation out of the way before I could deliver my son because it was blocking him from coming out. That was the only time I felt any discomfort. And, and that was just mainly because I was having to push when I didn't feel ready to push, necessarily. Like I was forcing a push when my body wasn't ready to. And so, I mean, anytime you try and do something like that, whether you go to the bathroom or not, it's kind of uncomfortable. So, then, but as soon as that was done, the rest was easy. I—most people have the, like the "ring of fire" when the baby starts crowning. I didn't have it ... I was holding him and I just it was so surreal like that it had happened that quickly. And that I'd actually got what I wanted. You know? I was just happy. I was elated. I was like, like, about 20 minutes after I had my son, I'm sitting there. And I looked at myself in the mirror. I was like, "I don't look like I just had a baby." (LAUGHS).

As a theme, preparation echoes throughout these birth stories, Araceli's included. During her first pregnancy, Araceli had been given information and a book about hypnobirthing, in her skepticism, "blew it off." In her view, the traumatic experiences that she had endured during her first birth had paved the way for her second ecstatic birth experience because they had planted within her the drive to find a different way. She dove into hypnobirthing this second time around, and in so doing, trained herself throughout her pregnancy for an entirely different birth experience in terms of meditative hypnobirthing practices and language. She protected both her head space and body space in new ways. Her second birth process transformed her mindset from one that upheld that others somehow have power over her birthing body to one that honors the power vested entirely within herself. In her words:

> ... so, we got there [to the hospital in labor]. Got the nurse. I put my headphones on. And aside from saying my name, "She's my representative," I did not talk to the nurses. I like completely ignored them. I just focused on all my visualizations and my like—And it was barely—really like, amazingly not painful. I cannot like, say, you know, how not painful it was. And when they examined me in their whatever triage table, they're like, "Oh, you're seven centimeters dilated." And I was like, "Yes. I know how to do this! I am powerful!" [LAUGHS]. I actually, I don't—I didn't know that at the time. But I knew I was doing my job. I think they had confirmation that I was doing my job.
>
> [Delivery] was really intense. Not—I wouldn't say horrible, but it was really intense. I loathe to say painful because I worked so hard to like—but it wasn't painful ... I turned over. And on that third sort of push—which you're not also supposed to do in hypnobirthing, you're supposed to just breathe through it—but I, like, at that point, I'm like "AHHH, I know how to do the pushing!" And like, I could feel the body of the baby. Like "There's the head!" And it was like I—I felt like—none of the other births, I could feel anything—I mean at one birth. But it's like "plop head, plop shoulders, plop butt" and that's like my—my—I could see—I could feel her like plop-plopping out of me. And I was ecstatic!

Overall, these pain-free births hold some consistent themes about the study participants' iterations of their pleasurable birthing experiences. The themes of head space, mental state, autonomy, power, and surrender, all come into play. And their abilities to enter into those spaces of power, surrender, and head space for many took rigorous preparation, specifically hypnobirthing, which is a specific set of techniques. However, I find it notable that some of these participants who'd had a pain-free birth had either expected it or had directly aimed for it, while others had not. I would also like to highlight that the study participants who reported these pain-free birth experiences span many racial identities and geolocations. I touch on this more in the coming section dealing with the sociocultural aspects of birth pleasure. Now, I move to an expansion out from this set of completely pain-free birth experiences to partially pain-free births without analgesia.

Partially Pain-Free Birth without Pain Medication

I've separated these births from those that I've described in the previous section because there had been painful aspects to these participants' birthing experiences that had gone far beyond momentary lapses in their head spaces or sudden flare-ups of fear. These births had, to varying degrees, involved complications such as tears, dilation issues, a coccyx injury at delivery, as well as the more typically socioculturally normalized pains that I've also described above, such as the infamous "ring of fire." However, these births were pain-free in many other ways, even in ways that had surprised and delighted the birthing person, such as contractions, transition, rupture of membranes, or even crowning and delivery being pain-free and without the use of pain-relieving pharmaceuticals.

Callisto gave birth for the first time at home at age 27 and described the sensations of her labor as not only having been "pain-free," but also as having been "arresting" in their intensity. In her words:

> I wouldn't describe it as pain because when I actually knew I was in labor, I was ecstatic (LAUGHS). I was like, "Oh, my god, yes! It's finally happening!" I didn't have to use castor oil. I didn't have to see the acupuncturist. My midwife was right. Um, I was actually just like, overjoyed. So, when I started, I felt them, but I wouldn't describe it as pain ... I wouldn't really describe it as pain. It was just more so just like, intensity, I guess. It was arresting and its quality, I guess ... So in thinking about pleasure, and how it impacted my postpartum, like my immediate postpartum, my birth was perfect. Like it was exactly except for tearing. That hurt. Except for that, the birth itself was great. My daughter was healthy. When she was born, she was alert. She was not crying whatsoever. And I was on an oxytocin high that was just out of this world!

Cande also experienced some painful aspects of their roughly 24-hour labor but still conveyed their experience of birth as mostly pain-free, and mainly just physically intense. Their first-and-only birth, they labored at home until things were quite far along, then transported to deliver at an autonomous birth center. This transport was one of the few times during which they felt very uncomfortable during their labor. Dealing with confinements or any restrictions of their movements led to pain—this included the car ride and during fetal monitoring upon arrival at the birth center. In the context of peak COVID-19 pandemic containment policies, the birth center restricted whom they could bring to the birth; just their partner and a doula were admitted. All of their care providers wore masks throughout their labor. Cande was very thankful when a healthcare worker at this birth center advocated for them to have the birth tub opened and acted as a steward for their birth experience. In their words:

> I had like a new nurse show up and like the new nurse was like phenomenal. She was like this little like Goddess that came in and like the angel watching over and like I don't know why there was the change. But she was like, "Nope, we're gonna do like wireless fetal monitoring. It's waterproof." She like convinced the staff there to open the birth tub. So, I was the first person to give birth in the birth tub since COVID had happened. So, they shut it down in March. I gave birth in August. And then she was just like, as if she had, she and I had worked together in a like—for an entire lifetime. Like everything that I could have thought I needed, she was already there with it.

I have already described Cande's birthing experience above, but here I add some particularly salient excerpts from our interview that convey the ways in which their labor was pain-free, how transport and confinement had stalled their labor, and what they had experienced instead of "pain" at delivery, sparing a birth injury to their coccyx. In their words:

> I was channeling the energies going like down and sort of like forcing the energies down. And I could physically feel what was going to be [my baby], like going through me and moving down the birth canal, which was a really cool feeling. And then right, as [my baby] was being born, my doula said it went from like, zero visibility to then all of a sudden, the head was out. There was no, like, "Okay ... We're counting ... Okay, a little bit more ... like push a little bit." It was like, zero to 60. He was born. The midwife was nowhere to be found. My nurse basically had to jump in the tub, because by the time like [the baby] came, there were three pushes, one for the head, one for like, the torso, and then the feet. And that was it. So super quick. When it was actually happening, there was like this relief, but then I also felt this weird pop

> and pain, which I found out later was because [my baby] came so fast, dislocated my tailbone and sprained it—moved a disc in my tailbone and pinched my nerve, which led to like the ball of nerves under the tailbone, which explained a lot of things postpartum. (LAUGHS) Yeah. But the actual birth, like, it was just like, I had moved from like, sort of like lying down in water to being up on the side, and then just out of nowhere, well, not out of nowhere, out of me (LAUGHS) [the baby] came. And like the nurse basically had to like jump in. Because we—nobody was expecting it. Like I hadn't seen the midwife since intake. Like she hadn't even checked on me. Because at that point, I'd only been at the birth center for like, six hours, I think, and everything sort of stopped when I got to the birth center. So, my contractions that were at, like, two minutes apart [at home], had jumped back out to like 10 to 15 minutes apart. And on the whole, like birth scale thing, I was like, four centimeters dilated at intake. And I think they said like 70% effaced and at station zero or negative one. I think I was negative one [station], something like that. But so, the midwife was like, "I got plenty of time, like I don't," like she just wasn't around. And so like, my doula had to run to go get the midwife. The nurse practically caught [the baby] as he was, like, came out swimming in the water. It was her first catch, also, which was like kind of cool.

This story is remarkable in how it shows the broad variety of sensations that are possible in a first birth. Cande's birth was not precipitous. Her labor lasted roughly 24 hours. But the pushing phase (which for some lasts for hours) was a matter of minutes. Their birth story also shows the impact of transport on the progress of labor. Cande spent just six hours at the birth center in all, due to the strong labor flow that she'd established during their early labor at home. In terms of this birth being pain-free, Cande's experience reiterates that any interference in the mental and physical state of the birthing person can be a major detractor of birthing people's ease. These (often routinized interferences) instigate pain or hardship. Toward the end of our interview, Cande said:

> … you can create pleasure in some of the most displeasurable moments. But you have to really know yourself. And I think part of being able to experience pleasure through childbirth was really getting to know, deep down like, who I was, and what was pleasurable for me, and how to navigate those realms instead of leaving my agency … I really had to take over and claim—and like reclaim my agency. And I think had I not, it wouldn't have been a pleasurable experience by any means.

Marion's birth was free of any outside interference and confirms in some ways this thematic finding. As my readers will already know, I chose to use Marion's story as the starting place of this book, but here I focus on how Marion's second birth had largely been pain-free without any pain-relieving pharmaceuticals. This was her first vaginal delivery, as her previous birth was an emergency cesarean. This was also her first out-of-hospital birth. She labored at home overnight and delivered at an autonomous birth center the following afternoon. One brief experience of pain that she reported during this labor had been a cervical pinching sensation. In her words:

> … nothing was hurting except for just cervical pinching. I could just feel her head right there and I could just feel it jiggling as I moved. And it felt really good. Just move my hips and just kind of feel that cervical opening. Like that felt really good! And it didn't feel super painful, and the contractions were like, just demanded my attention. They weren't painful. They just demanded my attention … And my strategy from the beginning was something my midwife had mentioned that she did with her babies, which was just counting your breaths out loud. There's just something to think about and something to do. And just each exhale, I would say, one with my exhale. And two with my exhale, and like the longest contraction I ever had was, like 13 breaths. And I thought "Alright, anyone can do this for like 13 breaths." And then towards the end, they didn't even last till 13 breaths. So, I kept counting, and then it'd be over. And I was like, "Oh, wow, that was easy!" … I'm in the shower [at home]. And then it's like—I'm making noises! And it's still not even hurting. But it's like—I'm feeling it. Like I'm jiving with whatever energy is happening, whatever rhythm is happening … I was in transition, basically. But I didn't even know it …. I was just drawn inward not—not panicked, not worried, not—not even really complaining. Like not—Yeah, I was just grateful. I could just keep thinking the whole time "This so great! I can't believe I get to do this this time." Like, "I can't believe I get to be in this this time." And, and not missing any of it and not like, you know, hearing about it later." Like "I'm experiencing every second and it's so great!" ... And so, then we went with my husband and my doula to the birth center. And they had the tub ready. And I walked down the hall and got in the tub. And then it was like, "Okay, maybe this is like kind of ouchie now." And but she was like, pretty much coming out. I didn't even know it. And then I started to like push, right as I got in the tub. And the midwives hadn't even come into the room yet.

Marion associated that "ouchie" feeling with the last bit of stretch at delivery in its intensity, causing her to feel a bit of fear. In her words:

> I was like, "I, okay, I just pushed and that felt like so strong. I feel like I'm gonna tear if I embrace that. So, do I need to slow this down? Or can I just go with it?" And she [the midwife] was like, "Oh, yeah, just go into that." And then, so, they never checked me. Um, I just was pushing, and they're like, "Sure, go for it." And I was like, "Okay!" She was out in like 10 minutes. And I didn't tear at all ... I was just like, so excited and happy with how good it felt at that point. Like there was no more pain after her head was out. The only pain I remember was that initial—that last bit of stretch and being nervous that I was gonna like explode because there was no stopping it. And I wasn't doing it. It was like, my body is doing this by itself. And a "I hope it knows what it's doing" sort of a thing that was like a little moment of panic, I guess.

For a first vaginal delivery, an out-of-hospital VBAC, Marion's story illustrates the surprising ease and speed with which a birth can happen. While her labor lasted around 18 hours, almost all of that time was spent at home. She delivered her newborn at the birth center within the hour she'd arrived. The birth center staff never checked Marion's dilation nor interfered with her physicality. And Marion maintained a committed and clear mindset: she wanted to fully experience birth and felt grateful for the opportunity. As she herself stated, this birth had been a "tremendously healing" experience for her.

Aleks had also experienced two previous cesareans when they planned their third and fourth births out-of-hospital. Their first out-of-hospital VBAC, at age 29, took place at an autonomous birth center. Their second out-of-hospital VBAC, at the age of 36, took place at home (so, an HBAC, or home birth after cesarean). It is this VBAC home birth that had, in certain respects, been pain-free. Aleks reported no pain during their early labor, at the rupture of membranes (something had been painful during their previous births). During their HBAC, they had also not experienced the "ring-of-fire" or pain during their delivery. In their words:

> I remember my wife being like, "Oh, what's that?" and I was like, "My water broke." And I never had my water break with my previous babies. They—it was it always had to be initiated by the physician. And then my last baby, you know, it broke by itself and was really

> painful. So, this was like, not painful at all. And I was like, really, it's really how pleasure began during labor, in a sense, because it didn't hurt. And it was happening. And I was just like, "Oh, we're in labor." And I called my—my doula. And I was like, "My water broke." And she's like, "Let's go!" (LAUGHS) she—(LAUGHS) and it just set this tone of like, this is gonna go; this is happening. And this is gonna—like—I'm gonna be in charge … When I was feeling a lot of pain, I remember being like, "Is there anything else?" She's [the doula's] like, "No, unfortunately, I didn't tell you this. But there aren't things we can do. It's just you and your pain, and you're going to handle it. You're almost there." And then, when the midwife checked, and I was only seven centimeters, it was to my doula that I looked and I was like, like, I didn't verbalize it. I was just fearful and, and she looked at me, I remember, it was a very sexy moment. And she was like, "Well, seven is just a number. So, like, let's see how you do," then "Seven is just a number. I wouldn't worry about it too much" … But when I needed her [the doula] exactly how I needed her, she took a very dominating position with me and, and I responded well to that, because when I give people permission to do that way, and to have sex with me that way, or be that way with me, you know, I respond to it really well. And it worked because my brain is used to that as a pattern from my BDSM [bondage, discipline, sadism, masochism] experiences, obviously. And so, she was excellent. Like, exactly … Even if it was just such a brief moment, because I delivered right after that. She carried me those last five minutes.

Most of these stories touch on the impact of support persons on the mindsets of the study participants. For Aleks, their doula had shown up exactly as they needed her to, to help to maintain Aleks's mindset and ground their full experience of their birth. In their words:

> … the baby's head came out. And I was really surprised. And I put my—my hand down there and I felt the head and I was like, "The head is out!" (LAUGHS). I was so happy. But like, I was so shocked because it didn't hurt!

What is typically depicted as the most painful thing that can happen to a birthing person—delivering a baby vaginally—had "shockingly" been pain-free for Aleks, and without any anesthesia. And Aleks's experience was among several that I've shared in this section to indicate this very real possibility. Aleks went on to describe the long-reaching impacts of their birthing experience:

> I think I rewired my brain for thinking about labor in a pleasurable way. And that—and in doing so, you know, reclaimed, like power that was taken from me in the first two births—that were really, really traumatic ... it's definitely changed my idea of looking forward to something like labor. Because I'm excited now! And before, the pain and trauma overpowered everything. Like it was first that you think about. And now it's like, like, I can't wait to do that again. And well, that's a huge shift (LAUGHS), you know? And it's pleasurable to think about it in the future, as opposed to being afraid. I have no fear. It's just anticipation. And you can only learn that from having given birth, you know, that way. I know, I know, not every home birth goes like that. And I know that mine might not even go like that, but just that I had that one experience is enough to be like, "Hey, like, I know what I'm doing." I trust my body more, you know.

This fourth birth shifted their perspective toward birthing in the future from a pain-focused and traumatized perspective to a perspective of anticipation and excitement for birth, self-trust, and an orientation toward pleasure.

Partially Medicated Pain-Free Birth

Most of the hospital births included in my dataset involved the use of epidural anesthesia but nevertheless had not been described by my study participants as "pain-free" birth experiences. Only Raquel had, during our interview, articulated her epidural use as an aspect of her pain-free birth experience. She had given birth for the first time in a hospital just about a month prior to our interview, and had a pleasurable, although somewhat troubled, birth experience due to concerns about fetal cardiac decelerations in her most recent check-in with her care team. Her sense was that she was in early labor when she was admitted for an induction. In her words:

> I guess that my body had probably already started labor like that day, and I just didn't really feel it or notice, which is why things progressed so fast. Like I was on like, the smallest dose of Pitocin. They had to, like, turn it off after a while. So, I think it—things had been going for a couple hours. And then I finally started to actually feel the contractions. I'm not sure why I didn't feel them before ... there wasn't any pain. Wasn't until I was there for, like, a couple hours on the Pitocin that I was like, "Oh, yeah, this is kind of painful, and I'm gonna start kind

> of bringing in those techniques that I learned from yoga," trying to, like, relax, and like, lean into it, and like, go towards the feeling and like, be open to it. Rather than kind of like clenching up and like, tensing against the contractions ... It almost felt like it's like a deep meditation, where I was, like, very separate from the rest of the world while the contractions were happening. And I, I guess, I'd say they weren't painful, but they were more just kind of a sensation than they were like something unpleasant.

Although Raquel had an epidural placed in preparation for a potential emergency cesarean for the continued fetal heart rate decelerations, she reported that when the care team checked her cervix just after the epidural was inserted, she was 10 cm dilated. They told her that she could push. Thus, Raquel reported having greatly enjoyed a relatively pain-free labor before the epidural had even been administered, and in spite of the Pitocin-driven induction process, for which most birthing people receive epidural analgesia. She was disappointed with the experience of epidural analgesia, which, she complained, had completely removed her ability to feel her pushing and delivery stages. But, in the end, she did not regret it, believing that she this was appropriate care under the circumstances. The main themes that I want to highlight in Raquel's story are the techniques that she had intentionally used to maintain a calm and a meditative mindset during her labor within this hospital setting, and her "silent labor," which is similar to Chandra's, as I described at the beginning of this section. Several of my study participants, including those who had given birth in hospitals, were in little to no pain during their early or even active labors. Labor is not always painful for first-time birthing people, and a big part of that is mindset, particularly the absence of fear, or better yet, a willingness to experience the sensations without deciding in advance that they are painful.

Summary

For the 12 study participants who experienced pain-free births (52%), in whole (7, for 30%) or in part (5, for 22%), their mindset, head space, intentional use of language, strategic involvement of support people, sense of agency, and non-interference were the most common themes to emerge from our in-depth interviews. Most participants rejected pain as an inevitability and affirmed other possible ways to experience the sensations that arose during birth. Most of these participants had, during our interviews, shared a sense that their active preparation and mindset determined the degree to which their birth experience was pain-free, regardless of the setting in which they gave birth. In sum, pain-free birth exists. It exists for first-time births. It exists for folx who have had cesareans previously. It exists in hospitals and birth centers and in homes. It happens to Black, Latine/x/a, White, and Asian people across gender identities and sexual orientations, and presumably most any kind of person one might think of. It is possible, even for people who have had traumatic birth experiences in the past. Pain-free birth is only one variety of pleasurable birth experiences that can be learned from rather than summarily dismissed as an anomaly. My hope is that my readers, birthing people, and birth practitioners of all kinds, will take note of these possibilities. My study participants revealed many powerful clues as to how to improve birth experiences can be improved, perhaps liberated from pain and fear, perhaps enhanced with pleasure and joy, by and for birthing people from many (if not all) walks of life.

4

MEDICALIZATION, DE-MEDICALIZATION, AND PRAXIS

This chapter explores medicalization, de-medicalization, and the kinds of pleasure that were derived in praxis, be it within the embrace of biomedicine or defiance of it. Over the course of my research, I have grappled with the questions of 1) who is defining birth and 2) how. Regarding the dominant definitions of birth, medicalization weighs heavily. The medicalization of birth has been defined in many ways in the scholarly literature, ranging from value neutral to highly critical and value-laden definitions, and ranging in scope from the micro-scale of individual experiences to the macro-scale of social and/or cultural processes (van Dijk et al., 2020). Because my study has primarily focused on individual birth pleasure experiences as situated within their respective contexts, I use Barker's (2008) useful definition of *medicalization* as "the processes by which an ever-wider range of human experiences come to be defined, experienced, and treated as medical conditions" (p. 21). Birth has certainly "come to be defined, experienced, and treated" as a medical event in the United States. However, for this study, it is not as simple as discerning where a given birth occurred, or if medical interventions were used. Being interested in research justice, I've analyzed medicalization in my dataset based on my study participants' mindsets toward their own births, how their mindsets changed over time, and with whom they placed decision-making power. The distinction I've drawn here is about the orientation of the birthing person toward or away from medicalization. This orientation seemed to have occurred along a spectrum.

I also saw the need to disaggregate birth setting and interventions from my analysis of medicalization. Medicalization was predictably more

DOI: 10.4324/9781003499428-5

formal within biomedical settings (hospitals) than in community settings (free-standing birth centers and homes). However, some participants' births in hospitals were very much "de-medicalized," a term that I use for those who actively resisted medicalization in how they exercised their autonomy, engaged with the institutional powers at hand, and experienced their birthing processes. And interestingly, some of the home births that I describe below involved considerably more medical interventions (foley bulbs, stripping of membranes, intentional rupture of membranes, urinary catheterization, medications, etc.), than some of the hospital births that I also describe below. A more nuanced analysis was necessary.

Birth setting and parity, however, are critical layers to consider and I address them briefly here. All of my interview participants reported experiencing pleasure in birth at some point in their birthing lives, but not every birth discussed in our interviews was considered a pleasurable one. In total, 74% of all births in my interview dataset (32 of 43 total) were reported as pleasurable (including all types of pleasure):

- 13 of 24 hospital births were reported as pleasurable (54%)
- 14 of 15 home births were reported as pleasurable (93%)
- 4 of 4 autonomous birth center births were reported as pleasurable (100%)

In terms of parity, the vast majority of first births had occurred in a hospital (16 of 23, for 70% of first births), compared to first births at home (5 for 22%), and first births in an autonomous birth center (2 for 9%). First births are generally understood to be more difficult than subsequent births. In my interview data, indeed first births were less likely to have been reported as pleasurable than subsequent births (regardless of the birth setting).

- 14 of 23 first births were reported as pleasurable (61%)
- 11 of 14 second births (78%)
- 3 of 3 third births (100%)
- 2 of 2 fourth births (100%)
- 1 of 1 fifth birth (100%)

To attempt to tease apart how parity might be impacting birth pleasure as compared to the birth setting, I also compared how many first births were reported as pleasurable by the birth setting:

- First births in hospitals: 8 of 16 were reported as pleasurable (50%)
- First births in homes: 4 of 5 were reported as pleasurable (80%)

- First births in autonomous birth centers: 2 of 2 were reported as pleasurable (100%)
- First births out-of-hospitals: 6 of 7 were reported as pleasurable (86%)

This figure of 50% of first births in hospitals as having been pleasurable comports with the above figure that 54% of all hospital births having been pleasurable (regardless of parity). For my interview participants, 86% of their first out-of-hospital births were pleasurable. This same trend had held across all parities: out-of-hospital births were much more likely to be pleasurable than hospital births (95% versus 54%). Qualitatively speaking, I also found the same—that home and autonomous birth center births were more pleasurable than hospital births in my interview data. Of course, given the limits of this study as a primarily qualitative and ethnographic one, more research is needed to further extend my findings. But my intention here is not to make any claims of representativeness across populations of birthing people, but rather to check for biases in terms of my analyses and to test my study's conceptual validity. While some might prefer to wave off pleasure in birth as a fluke of fortune, as a happy accident, or as the result of having had many births or not having had any complications or perinatal trauma—these data show patently otherwise, even if just across 43 births. It's a start. Now, having attended to these potentially confounding aspects, I further delve into my study participants' mindsets across the spectrum of medicalization, which I've categorized in Table 4.1.

Birth Mindsets Across a Spectrum of Medicalization

> I really didn't think that would happen to me.
>
> *(Romi)*

Romi's quote just above reveals a paradoxical aspect of the medicalized mindset toward birth. While she had heard about concepts such as

TABLE 4.1 The Spectrum of Medicalization: A Summary of the Interview Participants' Birth Mindsets

Participant mindset	*n*	*Pseudonyms*
Medicalized	6	Callie, Romi, Dalisay, Raquel, Malika, Debbie
Medicalized first birth(s) then de-medicalized for subsequent birth(s)	8	Skylar, Sankofa, Veronica (minimally medicalized), Marion, Araceli, Aleks, Melissa, Theia
De-medicalized	9	Semiramis, Chandra, Callisto, Cande, Nava, Bree, Venus, Pearl, Fabia

"ecstatic" or "orgasmic birth," she shared with me that she never would have predicted that *she* would experience the kind of life-changing pleasure that she had indeed experienced. Within a medicalized mindset that is focused on the biomedical control of both pain and complications, pleasure complicates the field of what is predictable, possible, or probable. She and five other interview participants viewed their births as medical events first and foremost. They experienced their births as somewhat pleasurable (in whole or in part) within their respective hospital settings. Medicalization had been necessary for some of these participants (such as for preterm labors or a transfer from an autonomous birth center to a hospital due to complications) and had been a preference for other participants. Their preference was based on their underlying belief that "that's what birth is"—a medically managed experience within a hospital. These births tended to involve more complications and, as such, a greater number of biomedical interventions. These participants' stories featured a great deal of detail as to the particulars of the biomedical management of their births within hospital settings. The kinds of pleasure in these births spanned the full typology that I've covered above, except sexual pleasure. Primiparas in this category attributed their pleasurable experiences to sufficient birth preparation, personalized care, an enjoyment of being centered in care, and witnessing inspirational teamwork among the hospital staff. Multiparas cited a general improvement in their birth experiences with each additional birth, which they understood as the result of having given birth more than once and the associated greater knowledge, higher self-confidence, and a deeper sense of agency. Some pleasures (physical but non-sexual) had intentionally been generated by these interview participants themselves or by their care teams through comfort measures and/or meditative practices during their labors. Other types of birth pleasure arose spontaneously and caught the birthing person by surprise. These surprises mostly involved the emotional, mental, and physical pleasure that had immediately followed their deliveries, which were described as overwhelming and profoundly impactful.

> I would never have another hospital birth no matter what.
>
> *(Sankofa)*

Eight of the multipara study participants experienced medicalized-mindset births within hospital settings, followed by de-medicalized subsequent births (within a variety of birth settings). Although it is certainly possible that many people have non-traumatic medicalized first births that they find both pleasurable and satisfying (as I've described above), those interview participants who'd shifted from a higher degree of medicalization to a lower degree of medicalization reported great dissatisfaction with what they'd felt had been an excessive degree of medicalization of their previous births. They attributed the over-medicalization to having been of a young maternal age, to their ignorance about birth care and their options or desires, or to a default understanding that birth is by definition a medical event. As a result of negative or traumatic medicalized birth experiences, these participants questioned their previous understandings of birth and set out to de-medicalize their subsequent births. This pattern firmly held for all eight people multiparas in this category.

In general, experiences of birth pleasure were connected to the birthing person's sense of sovereignty, agency, reciprocal trust, and egalitarian care relationships that placed primacy on the birthing person's uniqueness, knowledge, and abilities. These participants took pleasure in their choices about birth including the setting, who would support them, and how, relishing a sense of power, but "power with" or "power over others" and not an experience of others exercising "power over" them. In the coming section, I focus specifically and deeply on one unique aspect of birth pleasure that emerged from the de-medicalized birth experiences—the "pleasure of defiance," which is a gleeful push-back against the "power-over" experiences that many of these participants had negatively experienced during their previous births.

Nine interview participants actively de-medicalized all of their birth experiences, regardless of their respective birth settings. These participants had birthed in hospitals, birth centers, or in their own homes. I struggled with naming this group. Partly, I think that "nonmedicalized birth" would be suitable, but I am also careful to use such a term because it implies that the hegemonic medicalized current US birth culture had somehow been absent for some of my interview participants. But that would not be true. These participants had fully acknowledged that there is a default of medicalization from which they'd chosen to diverge. So, I herein I choose to maintain the "de-medicalized birth" distinction here to honor their work to actively disrupt this hegemony during their own birth experiences, without necessarily having had any previous negative or traumatizing birth experiences. Thematically, their pleasurable birth experiences had hinged on several shared factors: high-quality support, environmental ambiance. Also, birth head space emerged as an important theme, regardless of birth setting. Head space is a term I use in this study to denote the unique mental, emotional, and interoceptive state of the birthing person during labor. There were also many pleasures that came with the full ownership of one's birth process, setting, and care relationships (particularly for those participants who'd delivered at home). Some of these participants had also experienced the "pleasure of defiance," which is a special theme that I will now address in depth in the following section of this chapter.

The De-Medicalization of Birth as a Liberatory Praxis

Those who are currently reclaiming their births from biomedicalization are reclaiming them into the purview of their own power, thereby imbuing these births with their cultural identities, beliefs, and dreams. De-medicalizing birth involves, for some, a queering of birth, thereby freeing it from gendered ideologies, and birthing in defiance of cisheteronormativity. For others, de-medicalizing birth involved asserting a new/different power within their own gender identities, a specific type of pleasure that they may feel in their matrescence (Davis-Floyd, 2022; Orchard et al., 2023), within their emerging and unfolding motherhood/parenthood. For still others, it had been the throwing off of any external constraints, particularly oppressive gender norms, to step into the fullness of their own sovereignty. In total, 12 of the 23 interview participants had experienced at least one of these qualitative dimensions:

- "Fuck off" birth (Araceli)
- "Fuck you" birth (Aleks)
- "Wild woman/bad girl/bitch" births (Semiramis, Venus)
- "My way" births (Bree, Callisto, Fabia, Marion, Melissa, Skylar, Sankofa)

Births with "pleasure in defiance," as I have distinguished them here, tended to be home births or births at autonomous birth centers attended by midwives, doulas, or in the case of one participant, Fabia, no one. However, the hospital births with this quality of "pleasure in defiance" demonstrated some potent information about the transgressive implications of pleasure in birth. Perhaps none of the interlocutors demonstrated this theme of pleasure so richly as Araceli (a straight Latinx woman, age 36 and 39 at the times of her births, living in Oakland, California), who'd had a very protracted and traumatic first birth experience, and for whom her second birth had been a major healing event for her. Giving birth to her second child in the hospital had not been her preference but was dictated by her insurance and financial situation. She practiced hypnobirthing meditative strategies (Mongan, 2016) in preparation for her second birth, which she described as follows:

> I call the second birth my "fuck you all birth." Because it is not about you. It's about me. [laughs] Like [shakes head no] … it's not a "fuck y'all," it's a "Fuck-off Birth." Yes. "Fuck off." Everybody fuck off! [laughs] … I felt like a cat, who's like "fuck off." [laughs]

The laughter throughout her descriptions of her hypnobirthing experience emphasized the delight that she'd taken in this new head space, partly because it had been a major departure from the disempowered and overpowered sense of self that she'd negatively experienced during her first, more traumatic birth. This time, upon her arrival at the hospital, Araceli had headphones in loudly playing her meditative hypnobirthing material, already in a deep self-hypnotized mental state. She declined to interact with anyone besides her hand-picked support people. She ultimately had an incredible, largely pain-free but very intense and "super fun" birthing experience: "You know, it was super fun. Super fun. That is not what you tell people, right? You don't go around telling people that your birth is super fun. [Laughs]." Her experience had been so unusual within this hospital context that shortly after her delivery, a nurse had arrived to change her IV fluids bag, per protocol. In her brazen style, Araceli responded: " 'What the fuck are you talking about? I have no IV. I'm fine.' And it was great! Like, I was high for weeks after that." Her delight in having successfully defied the expectations around her was palpable throughout our lengthy and in-depth interview. It is a kind of pleasure that is specific to those who are currently challenging the hegemonic birth culture around them, and Araceli had done just that, despite her place of birth.

Others who shared this qualitative theme of pleasure but had given birth outside of the hospital context include Aleks, a White, agender birth parent, who felt a similar reclamation of power and delight during their third and fourth births. After their traumatic first and second births during which they'd been pressured to undergo cesarean deliveries in the hospital, they had an empowering experience of birthing in an autonomous birth center in New York at the age of 29, just before the COVID-19 shelter-in-place orders had commenced. Aleks said:

> Part of me continues to feel giddy about circumventing systems designed to make you fail at birth. You know, and so I like feel like I got away with something, which is ridiculous. And I like—I know that it's kind of, you know, silly and sad. But, but that I'm not sure who I'm saying "Fuck You" to when I think of my birth and look back on it, but it's this kind of like, you know, "We got to do it." "We did it." And no one can take that away from me.

And they carried this ethos into their next birth, in their words:

> She [the doula for their third birth at the birth center] changed my life anyway, I will forever be grateful because she was just like, "Why don't you just come full circle and feel even more confident in yourself and do it at home?" And then I was like, "Okay?"

This home birth experience, for their fourth birth, had experiential layers of pleasure that had fundamentally been grounded in their gender identity, the nuances of their relationship with their wife, and the special energy that emerges within one's own private space:

> The way I was delivering was just unapologetic. It was, like, strong. And it was, it was not the divine feminine. It was like, you know, the more contemporary version of like, someone empowered, you know, and … So yeah, labor hurt. The other thing was that the doula encouraged, and the midwife too, my wife to lift up the baby during contractions, like my belly, and that would help you know, them engage in the pelvis and stuff. And it was like this really pleasurable experience because when my wife and I touch we, we have more of like an electric sexuality, in a sense—it's like, extremely charged. And so, while all of these people are around, she and I—she was like, picking up the baby and like putting me—and I was naked. And you could see there's photos of this too, her holding me. It's a lot like our sex, in general, because of just our connection.

Their experience of birthing at home reshaped their perception of birth in an enduring way:

> In any case, it's definitely changed my idea of looking forward to something like labor. Because I'm excited now. And before, the pain and trauma overpowered everything. Like it was first thing that you think about. And now it's like, like, I can't wait to do that again. And well, that's a huge shift [laughs] you know? And, and it's pleasurable to think about it in the future, as opposed to being afraid. I have no fear. It's just anticipation. And you can only learn that from having given birth, you know, that way. I know, I know, not every home birth goes like that. And I know that mine might not even go like that, but just that I had that one experience is enough to be like, "Hey, like, I know what I'm doing." I trust my body more, you know.

Some of these study participants' births had more of a "wild woman/bad girl/bitch" quality to them, in particular the hospital birth of Semiramis. Semiramis (a mixed-race White and Middle Eastern womxn, living in the Bay Area of California), however, had demonstrated this theme of "pleasure-of-defiance" during her first and only birth within a hospital setting at the age of 22. She considered herself self-educated about birth and had labored throughout her early labor at home. When she went to the hospital, she was considered "wild" and noncooperative by hospital staff after she'd arrived. A Russian nurse, who had formerly been a practicing midwife in Russia, befriended her and became her doula of sorts. In her words:

> I read and I got really scared about some things, but I used that fear to kind of push me in the opposite direction—of learning more. Um, and so I already knew that I didn't want anyone to interfere. Unless I personally asked for it. I knew that being empowered to make my own decisions, even if even if I was like, a total bitch [Laughs], was going to make me feel like I could listen to my body. And so, I kind of like had this personal agreement that I don't care if people are going to judge me or, you know, whatever, I'm going to say exactly what I feel no matter what and not let anybody hijack my experience. [Laughs] ... And so regularly, the nurses would come in and try to like, strap me down on the bed to listen to the baby's heartbeat and stuff like that. I was like, "I know, you have other ways. You can't make me lie down. I'm not going to." And so, I was just really bossy. And like [Laughs], very determined to have it my way. And I think my husband was a little bit shocked, you know, his little bit like, "Whoa, this is—" you know, like, "You're supposed to be nice to these people." [Laughs] But what ended up happening is one really kind nurse who had been a midwife in Russia prior decided to befriend me and basically doula me in the hospital. She, I guess, talked to the other nurses and said, "Okay, we've got a wild one here. She's not gonna listen. So, I better just stay in there with her," you know, "if anything happens." And she actually regularly reminded me of like the mind-body connection and that I had the power and was able to do it. And she was just a Godsend. She was the sweetest thing.

This passage, in light of the laughter that her sharing provoked, demonstrates the delight of self-allegiance in defiance of institutional power. Semiramis had been clear that she was not going allow herself to be dominated by any outside interferences, and the result had ultimately been an incredible birth experience that inspired her to support others as a doula. The sensuality of her birth is palpable in her language, from pushing to her postpartum reverie:

> I just—it felt amazing [to push]. Like it was the best feeling to just push when I needed to and just—and it was intense. It was a really intense, glorious drive to like—you know. And then I definitely felt pleasure in that.

> And then when she was crowning, I felt what they call the "ring of fire" you know, just like this radiant, intense pleasure stretching opening like—it was beautiful. It was like this burning, amazing feeling and—and that is what got me through, you know her coming out … she got herself in perfectly, this little position so she could just kind of like, slip out, like slither out like a little snake. [laughs]. She's like, "Whoooop"—it was very quick. And I was done. And I didn't tear. And I when I was done, like immediately, I was like, "Wow, I could do that again!" Actually, I'd like to.
>
> It was like—kind of like a runner's high in a way, I guess. Like I've, I've run a couple of 5Ks and like at one point you start like, just going, because it just feels good to keep going. So, kind of like that, but more intense and different [laughs]. Um, and like, it also felt kind of like otherworldly, like spiritual or something. Like, like, like I was expanding. But like, not just physically, like there was just like this openness and like freedom.
>
> It's really hard to explain. It was sort of like a choir singing. [laughs] You know, just like, like, just the most beautiful—if it was a sound, and I'm a little bit synesthetic, like, I've always kind of associated taste with sound or feeling a sound or like various, like, different senses. So, I mean, it was like a choir singing in my body. [laughs]

Being "wild" was one of the ways in which pleasure showed up for Venus as well. Venus, who is a mostly straight White woman living in the Bay Area of California, gave birth at the ages of 28 and 31, both at home. At the time of our interview, it had been 19 years since her last birth experience, and yet her descriptions were crisp and nuanced. Here is her emphatic description of this: "wild woman" type of pleasure:

> What I loved is I had never accessed my wild woman like that. I was, you know, I just don't give a fuck! For the first time of my life. Honestly, like, it was just, it was so liberating. That was what I loved about it so much, I'd never felt that liberated. I just, I would like strip my clothes off. And I remember just walking around naked and just like, directing everyone not caring [laughs] you know? So liberating. It was very primal. And it was interesting for my husband too because he'd never seen like a woman, that primal. When I'd grab an orange and just (while making hand gestures smashing an orange in her fist), you know, super primal. [Laughs]. It was so great. I was like, "Oh, my God, everyone needs to experience this!" [laughs]

Giving birth at home twice gave Venus a sense of privacy, freedom, and spiritual connection that she highlighted as major factors in her experiences of pleasure during both of these home births. (I drew on those aspects of Venus's interview in the typology of pleasure above, specifically in terms of both sexual and spiritual pleasures.) In some ways, the wild/bad/bitch quality of these two home births had created enough space around her wherein she could experience birth fully and in a state of total autonomy and freedom. These pleasures had created other layers of pleasure for these mothers/birthing people. This is exactly the kind of pleasure that is opposed and suppressed by the biomedical structures that are designed to overpower and to control the birthing person and the birthing process (for multiple examples of these structures and for descriptions of how they work, see Davis-Floyd, 2022).

There were also those who had experienced many pleasures in having given birth "my way," who'd completely refused to surrender to any of the pressures around them to give birth in someone else's way (but without identifying the experience in terms of being wild/bad/a bitch). Callisto, Fabia, Bree, Skylar, Sankofa, Marion, and Melissa fit into this "my way" category, and had described their pleasurable birthing experiences with layered emotions, laughter, and delight. Below I share some excerpts from our interviews that best capture this defiant aspect of their pleasurable birth experiences.

Bree took pleasure in defying the constraining ideologies that she encountered during her preparation for giving birth to her first child at the age of 25 and at home. She, a straight Vietnamese woman living in Utah, had decided that her birth was going to be pain-free. She invested both her time and her energy preparing for a pain-free birth by using hypnobirthing as a framework. She reported a completely pain-free experience of this first birth and with a tremendous amount of pleasure physically and emotionally. But the aspect of her story that taps into the "pleasure-in-defiance" category had emerged here in her words:

> I had a lot of naysayers. Throughout my pregnancy, when I had mentioned that I was going to be giving a natural birth and without any medical intervention—I was going to be doing a home birth at that, too—I had a lot of naysayers. And people just didn't believe that it was possible. And they said, you know, would try to tell me their personal stories or somebody else's story that they heard. And for me, I was just confident that I was gonna be able to do it on my own. I didn't really let those people bother me because their opinions don't matter. I knew I was going to do it. And I did it. And so, I remember, you know, after the birth, I was like, "I'm so excited to write about this or share my story," because I kind of just like, want to wave it in people's faces! The people that didn't believe in me, and didn't think that it was possible. So, I just have a lot more confidence in myself and knowing that my

> intuition never fails me. And I really am more adamant about sticking to my beliefs, even though they may be unconventional.

Callisto (a straight Black woman living in Urbana, Illinois, who gave birth for the first time at home, age 27) spoke about having claimed her own realm of power and the impact of birthing in her way:

> You don't really have to involve a whole lot of people in your birth or your pregnancy, because you and your partner, or you and whoever, who are responsible for conceiving that child, and so it's not really, you know—I heavily discourage people from taking advice from the peanut gallery. Because I'm not going to go and talk to Joe Blow in the supermarket about my ability to achieve orgasms. So why would I talk to him about my child's gender? ... having a bedroom kind of mentality in terms of "This is my birth; this is my body; This is my private business." ... I birthed exactly the way I wanted to, minus the hemorrhaging. So yeah, I think—I think oxytocin and pleasure went a long way ... I think birthing the way that I wanted to has allowed me to be confident in myself, and making my own decisions about myself, and my body, and my children.

Callisto's experience of pleasure in birthing "my way" was partly in defiance of the hegemonic birth structures she refused to be subjected to, and in part about race and the entitlement that she'd experienced to her body and her child's body within "White spaces." I draw on Callisto's powerful observations of how racialized spaces impact experiences of pregnancy, birth, and postpartum in the following section addressing race. But for this "defiance" theme, it is clear that she'd derived a specific flavor of pleasure in having defied what she'd perceived as invasive power dynamics and structures during this first birth, and birthing "her way" had been both a reclamation of her own power and a declaration of her own sovereignty that carried her forward into her mothering journey.

Similarly, Melissa, a straight, mixed race Black and Latina woman, living in Brooklyn, New York, had also birthed for the first time at the age of 19 in a hospital and at home for her second birth at age 32. She expressed a similar sense that birthing in her way, what she called a "personalized birthing experience" had been fundamental for her mothering identity going forward, saying that it had "laid the foundation for a new child-rearing experience." During our interview, she expanded upon this theme as having contributed to her decision to devote herself entirely to mothering:

> When my [hospital-born] daughter was coming up, I was constantly "Am I doing this right? Am I like scarring her life?" It's—you know, I—it's just that constant self-doubt. But, you know, managing my pregnancy, having that childbirth [at home], being able to make this plan, and it come to fruition, just made me more secure in my decisions, I guess, as a parent. And I never wanted many children after my daughter. I didn't want any more children. And now after this [second] experience—I'm 34—so I told my husband like, "If there's any way we can get 10 kids in the next two years, we should do it, we should just go for like triplets two more times, and we'll be good." But now I want—I want a lot more children. And I just, you know, I want to—I just want to be a mom. Really-really. I've had this career. When I was 21 years old, in construction management. Very stable, sturdy, secure, lucrative career. And that means nothing anymore. All I want to do is just be home with my family. People think I'm crazy.

This sense of the life-shifting impact of birth itself was also echoed in Marion's interview. I have discussed her experiences at length in the Introduction to this book, but for this particular theme of pleasure, Marion's story highlights the "my way" dynamic of birthing sovereignty as a gateway to mothering and parenthood, and also the transformative differences in impact between environments of control versus those of support. All participants who'd experienced "pleasure in defiance" have shades of this sentiment that ultimately there is so much to gain and to lose in the moments of birth, and for these participants, having experienced self-sovereignty had been paramount to their experiences of pleasure in birth, and to their journeys into parenthood/motherhood.

Lastly, I want to present some of the thoughts of a midwife whom I interviewed about her unattended childbirth experiences. Fabia, a straight White Spanish woman living in the United Kingdom, gave birth to her two children at the ages of 33 and 35, and both of these births had occurred in her own home, completely unassisted by any other professionals or support people, in what some call "freebirth." Whereas her pleasure in the actual birth space itself had not been specifically expressed in a sense of "defiance," her choice of birth setting and her approach were by definition defiant of the biomedicalized hegemonic birth culture. At the conclusion of our interview, Fabia offered this critique from her perspective as a midwife practicing in hospital settings:

> It's quite silly how we have come to the point where we ask someone who doesn't know us how we are. Like when you go to the doctor to the—he sees you for three minutes, and it's "Is everything okay?" How is that possible that we've completely moved so far away from our own body? ... [As a midwife providing care in the hospital] When I can see, with all the technology, that everything is going fine, and the woman tells me it's not, I'm very, very cautious. Because, well, who knows your body better than yourself? So, I think they [birthing people] just need to own it. And they just need to know that your body is yours. Your birth is yours. And the only way to have a pleasurable experience is to own that experience.

Fabia drew my attention to embodiment as being core to birth sovereignty. She wants all birthing people to know their own bodies and that their births are theirs. And indeed, the de-medicalized birthing experiences as I've described above by some of these study participants show the ways in which birth is currently and joyfully being reclaimed. They are those giving birth with their own writhing energies. Their stories embody wildness, both its equanimous quiet and its untamed roaring. They birth sloppily and unapologetically. They birth within a beloved's tender gaze, in an intimate darkness or in a sparkling light, with sensuous or titillating touch. They give birth in their own uncontrollable unfolding. These interviews show how some childbearers are bringing forth life on their own terms, with their own hands and with their whole selves, and they tell us all that it feels amazing.

Summary

The spectrum of medicalization that I've explored throughout this chapter spanned both medicalized and de-medicalized birth mindsets, including those who'd traversed between these two perhaps polar spaces. Medicalized births often involved pleasures associated with the birth setting but tended to be articulated as either the alignment of the birthing person with the medicalized space wherein they birthed (having been centered by their care team, for example), intentionally generated through comfort measures (such as massage) or endogenous pleasurable experiences that caught the birthing person by surprise, not fostered by their birth setting or aligned with their medicalized orientation toward birth. Their experiences had included every type of birth pleasure except for sexual pleasure.

De-medicalized births involved all of the types of pleasure, including a distinct variety of pleasure that I named above: "pleasure in defiance." This particular kind of pleasure was experienced by many of my study participants who'd actively chosen to resist hegemonic birth culture and to reclaim both their own power and agency. From the "fuck-off" feel of Araceli's hospital hypnobirthing experience to Alek's unapologetic "Fuck you" home birth, to Semiramis's unleashed "wild/bad/bitch" hospital birth, to Callisto's take-no-nonsense "my way" home birth, these study participants have collectively painted a picture of how fun, joyful, and empowering birth can be whenever the sovereignty of the birthing person is centered by their care providers. This sovereignty had made other birth pleasure experiences possible for these interview participants. Those who'd engaged in the de-medicalization process had demonstrated a praxis, a path toward transforming this, again, presently hegemonic and heavily biomedicalized birth culture within the burning cauldron of childbearers' lived experience. "Pleasure in defiance" fueled birthing people in ways that had extended far beyond their births, far out into their futures, and into their parenting identities and also far beyond these. The interview participants whom I've presented herein also shared a desire to spread this knowledge, to share their insights with others. Because "praxis" is a reflective and a reflexive approach to shifting social norms and even cultures through birthing people's lived experiences (Bolaza, 2020; Cheyney, 2008), the births that these study participants described had indeed been aligned with this notion of praxis for social change.

References

Barker, K. K. (2008). Electronic support groups, patient-consumers, and medicalization: The case of contested illness. *Journal of Health Social Behavior*, *49*(1), 20–36. https://doi.org/10.1177/002214650804900103

Bolaza, E. B. (2020). Birth pleasure: Meanings, politics, and praxis. *Journal of the Motherhood Initiative for Research and Community Involvement*, *11*(1). https://jarm.journals.yorku.ca/index.php/jarm/article/view/40595

Cheyney, M. J. (2008). Homebirth as systems-challenging praxis: Knowledge, power, and intimacy in the birthplace. *Qualitative Health Research*, *18*(2), 254–267. https://doi.org/10.1177/1049732307312393

Davis-Floyd, R. (2022). *Birth as an American rite of passage* (3rd ed.). Routledge.

Mongan, M. (2016). *HypnoBirthing: The Mongan method*. Souvenir Press.

Orchard, E. R., Rutherford, H. J., Holmes, A. J., & Jamadar, S. D. (2023). Matrescence: Lifetime impact of motherhood on cognition and the brain. *Trends in Cognitive Sciences*. https://doi.org/10.1016/j.tics.2022.12.002

van Dijk W., Meinders, M. J., Tanke, M. A. C., Westert, G. P., & Jeurissen, P. P. T. (2020, August). Medicalization defined in empirical contexts – A Scoping Review. *International Journal of Health Policy and Management*, *9*(8), 327–334, PMID: 32613806. https://doi.org/10.15171/ijhpm.2019.101.

5

THE SEXUALITY CONNECTION IN PLEASURABLE BIRTH

How does sexuality affect birth? How does birth affect sexuality? These interrelationships are the focus of this chapter, specifically addressing sexual orientation and gender as sociocultural aspects of birth. First, I analyze the role that sexuality played in labor and birth, focusing on those participants who had sex during early labor or just before labor had started. Then, I move through the remaining three themes that emerged in the in-depth qualitative interviews with regard to how birth pleasure related to sexuality going forward after birth: (1) personal sexual empowerment; (2) physiologic changes; and (3) relational factors. Then, to expand the lens both outward and inward, I consider my study participants' sexual orientations and gender identities, important aspects of both self-knowing and relating, and the pleasures that connected to these aspects of their identities.

The Impacts of Sexuality on Labor and Birth

Some of my interview participants felt that there was a strong connection between their sexuality and the pleasure that they experienced during birth, and others not at all. First, a nod to those for whom sexuality was not salient. "I don't think there's anything that comes to mind on that topic" had been Raquel's response. For her, sexuality and birth had not been connected at all. Veronica had taken my question about sexuality to be more concerned with her relationship with her husband. Her thoughts:

> I guess in terms of intimacy at least, that wasn't really a foundational part of either of my labors. Like, one of my pleasures was not some

DOI: 10.4324/9781003499428-6

> kind of, like, beautiful connection with my husband. You know? The first time I think he had a little bit of like a deer-in-the-headlights and wasn't sure what to do. And then the second time, he was basically like, my pool boy [Laughs].

Here Veronica, rather comically, has provided an example of where her sexuality (at least in relation to her husband) had not at all been a salient part of her birth. The sexuality questions occurred as beside the point or completely irrelevant to her pleasurable birthing experiences.

Leaning a bit more toward sexuality in birth, Semiramis connected the closeness and intimacy that she'd felt with her husband with the many kinds of pleasure that she'd experienced during her first and only birth:

> I think that probably the closeness and intimacy between my husband and I, during the birth, helped a lot. Like, we danced a lot. He petted me and held me, and I directed him, and he listened. So, that intimacy was really important during the birth, for sure.

However, their relationship ended shortly after this birth. A longer-range connection between her pleasurable birth experience and her sexuality had not been salient for Semiramis. She felt more that the birth had been its own internal experience during which she'd felt "empowered" and "unleashed." She held these feelings as distinct from her sexual evolution, as it had taken a bit longer for her to develop a sense of autonomy and power around her own sexuality after this relationship had ended.

Next, I focus on those for whom sexuality played a more direct role in their birth experiences. Four of my study participants, Nava, Venus, Cande, and Pearl, engaged in sexual activity just before labor started or during the earliest stages of their labors. Their sense of the relationship between sexuality and birth is in some ways distinct. I have already described many of their pleasurable birthing experiences in detail in the "Sexual Pleasure" section of Chapter 2 on the typology of birth pleasure. Here, I focus on Pearl's interview. Pearl spoke at length and with great clarity about how sex, her sexual relationship with her partner, and her own relationship to her sexuality impacted her birth process during her first and only home birth. Pearl had experienced roughly four days of prodromal labor and had quickly been approaching 42 weeks of gestation, and so Pearl and her husband had sex to attempt to spark labor.

> With the prodromal labor, we had sex maybe on the like four days before because I was a week and a half late, like late quote-unquote, past the due date. So, we were like trying to rev things up ... the day

> before [the birth], the contractions were really intense. So, I wanted to have sex and like get into my body and also just a different head space. And so, we did, and it was really profound. It felt very intense. It was erotic. But my mi—I think my body took over so much that it shut my mind off a little bit more. Um, and so I felt like I was able to go into in different depth with intercourse then I feel like I had been before. And feeling those huge contractions and then orgasming felt just massive. It just felt like a very, very deep, carnal space to get to.
>
> I remember I definitely initiated because I didn't feel aroused, or like horny, or like, "Come on, baby," like, "I want this." It was more like "I need to shift—I want to shift what I'm feeling." And like, "Gimme something." [laughs] And so I desired exploring to see if sex would shift it. And so, I definitely initiated and make a note of some foreplay. But I wanted more intensity. Because I wanted to match the intensity [of the contractions] in some way.

Although Pearl's sexual experiences had not translated into an "orgasmic birth" in that the contractions had not been orgasmic in sensation, from there on out, Pearl believed that the sexual experiences she had early in her labor helped her deepen into her own unique birthing head space:

> It wasn't intellectual. There was just a very felt experience of going that deep without having any rational thought process, you know? I felt like my brain was totally turned off. And so, that was amazing. It helped the process. It helped to sort of ease the pain, I guess, or shift the pain. And make a really good connection too, with my partner.

She was able to move through her labor without going into a fearful head space, which she attributed to her sexual and spiritual work. Over the years she'd become familiar with pain and how to surrender into intense experiences, particularly sexual ones. This ability is something that she'd consciously named as a privilege:

> I did dominatrix work for about five years. And I feel like that also helped me a lot—and I never would have connected the two. But I don't like pain. I don't get off on pain. But in those spaces, I often switched [to a submissive role] just to experience the other side. And so, it was interesting, because I experienced a lot of things with other female Dom friends who would like try things out. And it was a very fun, playful space. So, I feel like it was interesting too, because I got into a lot of

> physical spaces that were not comfortable. To the point of painful. And it was interesting, because in those experiences, I feel like I allowed myself to not be triggered by it, or I was able to let go of my head and just like experience it. Because it was in a safe space, a consensual space, whatever it might be. And even though it didn't give me pleasure, it allowed me to experience it physically. So, I think that it actually helped me a lot. Just allowed me to get into my body more, I think.

Pearl had also discussed past psychedelic experiences that she believed helped her to learn about how to surrender control and to gain familiarity with altered states of consciousness:

> I'm really curious about psychedelics. And so, I did ayahuasca with the intention of getting rid of shit that I don't need that I'm subconscious about, you know? I can actively work on breaking cycles of my mom or like breaking the cycles of this—working on trauma or assault that I've experienced. But I was like, "Whatever I'm not aware of, I want to see if I can like shift it so that I'm not passing things on," you know, as much as I could. It was kind of my own experience. And that was really intense. And I think that allowed me also to let go of control, and trust that when I do let go of control, things are okay, if not better. Even though there's a lot of physical intensity and like getting to a space [in birth], like losing your cognitive reality—it is something that I feel like I've experienced in psychedelic spaces that helped me consciously kind of get to that place with birth. Because you do lose elements. You shift. Your cognitive state shifts, you know? And I feel like I was able to just sink into it more ... I feel like I come from a privileged space and being able to experience those things and like moving into pregnancy and birth with those understandings.

Previous work Pearl had done around sexual shame had also freed her up to experience many types of pleasure during her birth:

> I think a lot of times we really separate motherhood and sexuality, or our pregnant bodies and sexuality, or our postpartum bodies and sexuality. So, I think just cognitively I don't have that bias, or judgment or shame around it. So, I felt very free to be like, "Yeah I'm totally pregnant and really enjoying this right now," you know what I mean? Like, with this baby about to pop out, and I can fully sink into this without feeling any, like perverseness or anything like that. So, I think that also has helped.

Pearl is also a doula, and so her familiarity with the birth process helped her to be free of fear during her own birth experience.

> I'm a doula, as you know. I trained as a doula, so I feel like I was aware of a lot of the birth process ahead of time, too. So, the fear—even though you get the information, your lived experience can still be very fearful. But I felt like it helped ease my fear.

Overall, Pearl is one example of an interview that had gone into great depth about how sex and sexuality had shaped her birth process. Again, the theme of "head space" has emerged here as being paramount to both birth pleasure and to sexuality, as a tool to get there for some people, particularly for someone who is very connected to their sexuality. What had been more common among the interview participants and had also been shared with me by Pearl had been the sense of empowerment, the physiologic changes, and the relational changes that improved their sexual lives after their pleasurable birth experiences. There were also those who reported the opposite—that their sexual lives during their postpartum periods had been much more difficult or less satisfying, mostly for physiologic and relational reasons.

The Impact of Birth Pleasure on Sexuality

Empowerment

Most participants had experienced their pleasurable births as empowering, particularly in the ways in which they are now living their sexual lives. Part of this trend was a new sense of their bodies, new respect and appreciation for their bodies, and a new understanding of how powerful they are. Another aspect was a sense of increased freedom and facility with the body, through understanding and trusting the body more. This aspect is connected to their relationships with themselves as well as to their partners' relationships with their birthing bodies (I expand on this aspect further below in the relational section of this chapter.). Many of these study participants had also shared with me their increased sense of empowerment in the face of the sexist, misogynist, and the sex-negative societal/cultural ideas about sex and the female body. This kind of empowerment had greatly helped them to heal from their past sexual trauma(s), and to re-gain hold of their "authentic sexuality" as Chandra had put it, and, as Debbie had also described it, their sense of "sexual autonomy."

Pearl had brought a great deal of her personal sexual power and awareness to her first birth, and shared that in the end, her birth experience sexually empowering, within a sort of feedback loop. She'd also told me that: "Giving birth was an empowering experience that I feel translates into my sexuality for sure." But now, I ask: in what sense is birth empowering? The main ways in which these pleasurable births had been viewed as having been so empowering had to do with these participants' improved relationships with their bodies. For example, Bree had used her memory of her birth experience as a mental anchor to get herself back into a positive relationship with her body whenever she feels self-critical or negative:

> Every day in my life, and you know, anytime I have any negative feelings about myself, I just have to step back and think like, "Hey, you have an amazing daughter, and you gave birth to her and your body's amazing, it's capable of amazing things. So why are you hating on it?" I feel a lot more empowered.

For some of these study participants, their relationships with their bodies have greatly improved as the result of having experienced birth pleasure, and in turn this has improved their sexual relationships. Bree had continued during our in-depth interview:

> I just feel like I have a new—new sense of sexuality. I'm more comfortable with myself, and how I'm able to perceive myself in those ways. Before it was kind of like shameful ... I felt kind of ashamed of how my body looked or what it was. But now I feel very empowered with my body because of this whole experience.

For Sankofa, knowing her own embodied power and having that power witnessed by her husband has deepened their sexual connection and sense of control over their reproductive lives. This sense of reproductive control has led to less worry and more pleasure:

> I think, for me, I think it [sex] got better, actually. Just knowing, especially after the home births, knowing how strong and powerful my body was having my husband witness that, I think that heightened things. I think, also, for me, because I practice the rhythm method and herbal birth control, when I finally delved into that and got that almost down to a science, sex was more pleasurable for me, because I wasn't always worried about like, "Gosh, am I gonna conceive?" That whole thing really will inhibit you, you know? [laughs]

Self-trust, particularly trust in one's own body, was a major aspect of this bodily empowerment, and, for Marion, it translated into other aspects of early parenting, as well as having greatly contributed to her new sense of heightened sexual satisfaction:

> I feel like I'm whole, I guess. It feels like I can trust my body, the trust in my body, in "Whoa, pushed by itself, and it knew what to do, and I just had to go with the flow." And that's really carried on through like breastfeeding and stuff. We had some hiccups in the beginning, but I was just like, "I'm not gonna pump. I'm not gonna worry about my supply. I just trust that my body's doing it, even though I can't really understand." And it was. She was getting milk the whole time, even though I thought I had nothing [laughs], you know? And yeah, it just carried over with trusting my body. Our sex life has gotten SO much better since birth, I'm not sure if that's just hormones, but I'm good with it.
>
> And it's just like this trust of my body, I guess. And whatever is happening. I'm not analyzing my noises. I'm not analyzing the way I look. I'm not analyzing anything. It's just very spontaneous. We're having a blast together. He's just like my partner in fun. And that is—I think a lot of that does come from the birth experience, and just like, trusting what's happening, trusting me.

Marion, Bree, and Sankofa have brought together the ways in which sexuality is impacted by birth pleasure. They'd collectively described these as "a shift in their relationship to their embodied selves." Birth is experienced at every level of the self, but the very ground of the birth experience is obviously the body. For them, when their relationships with their bodies had shifted, everything else had also shifted, including their deeply embodied sexualities. Another aspect of empowerment that had often been highlighted during these interviews had been about how their births had empowered these participants in the face of oppressive ideologies such as sexism, misogyny, rigid gender roles, sexual shame, and past trauma(s). Debbie had reclaimed her body from the sexist and misogynist ideas that her body belongs to men:

> After giving birth, I began to see my body as more belonging to me to do with as I wanted, and to engage in sexual activity for me, versus for a man, to meet a man's needs. So, in a very subtle way, I would say it's that empowerment piece, it's that moving into your own body piece, that accepting that you own—that you live in your body. That kind of got turned on, that switch.

During our interviews, both Dalisay and Semiramis had sadly mentioned having experienced childhood sexual shame. Dalisay had spoken about her youth and her relationship with sexual pleasure, and about having refused traditional Filipina gender roles as a young adult, which she'd closely connected to her freedom to experience sexual pleasure later in her life:

> I think, you know, like that kind of—discovering my sexuality and, and moving away from all of those gender roles, and then Catholicism may have to go hand in hand. If I'm gonna pursue one, I have to shun the other. And I haven't turned back to religion since then.

Semiramis had highlighted that she'd never felt any shame about experiencing pleasure, which she'd connected to her ability to feel pleasure during her birth experience:

> I never felt shame about pleasure, which is interesting. Like I, starting at age like 12 or 13, I like started masturbating and stuff like that. And I never felt like it's bad for me to feel—to get to know my body in this way.

Callisto had also spoken about sexual shame and about her practice of dismantling it:

> I think sexuality and birth are related because there is a lot of like, guilt and shame that happen around both, and just mothering in general. And I feel like that's the underbelly of those things. And I think my personal mission is to be free of guilt and shame in everything that I do. And to me, that means being informed, and consenting, and being, you know, just aware of the consequences of what I'm doing.

She, a Black woman, explicitly named that her total sense of empowerment and ownership of her birth experience was founded on a deep "Black feminist analysis" of the body and on a commitment to live unencumbered by the thoughts and ideologies of others:

> I feel like where my sexuality is concerned, the way that it affected my birth experience is that, you know, I was reading and listening to things that reinforce the idea that you don't really have to involve a whole lot of people in your birth or your pregnancy … I think that not only having a private and intimate birth setting, which was my home, which was with my husband and choice people that were like cherry-picked to be there … just kind of added to the notion that this really isn't everybody's concern or everybody's business despite what society might tell you and despite how women are treated that, you know, especially women with children are treated.

During our interviews, Chandra and Theia had also shared with me about having sexually traumatic pasts, and that their birth experiences had helped them to regain themselves and their sexual self-awareness. Chandra credits her births with this re-evolution:

> So having them [my children], and the process of having them and raising them helped me to learn about my body, to learn what my authentic sexuality was, and helped me to demand it. Not settle. All of that came through from having my kids.

Theia has discovered that, since giving birth, she has been more able to be true to who she is, including having ultimately discovered her authentic sexual orientation:

> I have some trauma history. So that makes intimacy pretty difficult. So yeah, and since all of this [birth experiences], I am in a place now where I'm comfortable enough. I'm being true to who I am. And I'm finding out that I don't—I am not good with males and females are better for me. And so, I think that makes a difference as well.

Debbie had beautifully summed up how her journey through birth, as difficult as it had been for her, had completely and positively changed her sexual life: "My children definitely made me more sexually empowered and sexually autonomous." Overall, "empowerment" has been an important theme that had frequently emerged when, during our interviews, we'd discussed the interrelationship of birth with the participants' sexualities. They had shared with me all about how their relationships with their bodies had dramatically changed and in positive directions, and that this newfound sense of self had also greatly contributed to their self-confidence, joy, and self-expression in their sexual relationships. These participants had also relayed a newfound ability to be true to themselves in the face of the various oppressive sociocultural ideologies that have strongly and negatively impacted their sexuality, including sexism, rigid gender roles, sex negativity, and sexual shame.

Physiological Changes

Interview participants raised the physiological changes that they'd experienced during their pleasurable births as having been closely related to their sexual lives going forward, in positive, mixed, and negative ways. In this section, I address each of these three ways, starting with the positive ways.

Positive Impacts

Several interview participants reported that their sex lives had become better, in many cases much better, since their pleasurable births. Skylar, for example, had compared how orgasmic she'd been before having a baby to how she feels since: "It [orgasm] was rare. It was rare beforehand. Um. But after now, it's extremely, extremely orgasmic every time." Now this may strike my readers as surprising, because in general, the cultural narrative about postpartum bodies is that they are sexually dysfunctional, damaged, undesirable, uninterested in sex, or incapable of enjoying it. The actual physiological changes that occur during pregnancy and birth aside, participants named the impact of narratives about postpartum bodies as harmful. Postpartum bodies are often socially constructed as being loose, disgusting, unappealing failures that do not meet the standards of sexual desirability that idolize virginity-related qualities. Narratives that range from "getting your body back" to doing something about being "stretched out" or "wrecked down there," abound in the US, thereby negatively affecting birthing peoples' care choices. Some of my study participants had named these negative narratives and how they'd intercepted and/or countered them in their sexual lives. Bree had been very passionate in how she'd discussed these negative narratives:

> I think maybe women might be a little bit more self-conscious [sexually] because they gave birth. So, obviously, you're not the same down there. Or maybe they don't feel the same down there. So, I know that before I gave birth, I was a little worried about that. Because people talk about that all the time. "Oh," like, "You're a little bit looser," and "It's not as tight, so it's not as enjoyable for the man." So, I think that was a really big misconception because I've asked my husband, he says "No, like it feels the same—feels the same to me. Doesn't feel any looser or anything." So yeah, that's the biggest misconception.

Marion had also contended with the narratives and sociocultural ideas about what "having a good sex life" means with a postpartum body, which, as I've briefly mentioned above, is presumably not sexually desirable, is unappealing, and is thought to be sexually dysfunctional:

> I think my husband kind of always thought the opposite [that the pregnant and postpartum body is sexy], but it took me a while to like, trust him, I guess. Because I mean, I had stretch marks eight months into our marriage, boom. And I'm postpartum now. And I'm leaking milk now. And like, how does that relate to us having a good sex life? And

> I kind of had to integrate that. And he's been into it the whole time. It took me a while to believe him, I think.

In these ways, Bree, Skylar, and Marion had highlighted that sex can improve postpartum for some people, and that some of the barriers to this improvement are the negative cultural and/or social narratives that circulate around postpartum sexuality. Still, these three study participants had not reported having experienced any injuries during their births. Other participants had, indeed, experienced birth injuries. Those injuries had not always impacted their sexual lives in permanently debilitating ways. Even some interview participants who navigated birth injuries happily reported improved sexual experiences in the postpartum period.

Narratives about the postpartum body are rooted in the socio-cultural idea that delivering vaginally damages the vagina and vulva. Although, of course, birth injuries do happen, and I address this topic below, the matter is more nuanced. These interviews had completely made it clear that not all birthing people who deliver vaginally are injured or are negatively impacted by their birth experiences. Several of the participants, even those who'd experienced birth injuries, had also experienced an expansion of their abilities to experience multiple types of sexual pleasure in different ways. Some participants had connected this expansion to the physiological changes in their bodies. Pearl, for example, had experienced a small tear that had needed to heal, but when she'd finally returned to having sex with her husband, she'd been quite surprised by how "incredible" her sexual sensations felt:

> I had a small tear, but nothing that had needed stitches. The healing process was generally really solid for me. She [the midwife] came back a lot and checked in. So that also felt really held. And I think it was partially the connection that I had with [my husband] that six weeks after I was like, "Let's go!" like, "Can we go? ... Is it ... [Laughs] ... harmful in any way?" And he was so down. And it was amazing. And I felt like it was easier for me to get out of my head and into the sex space that we were in than ever before. And I also felt like, and I don't know how this is physiologically, what's up, but I feel like my G-spots have shifted, or are like bigger or something. And penetration feels better. Or not better—but like in a different intense way. So, I don't know, physiologically something has shifted, or if I'm just simply able to get there easier? So that was a huge thing ... If I had a very different birth experience, without as much pleasure—I don't know. Maybe it would still be super solid, but it feels like that definitely was a continuation of what got started in the birth phase.

Venus had also experienced a tear, in her case a severe tear that had required a hospital trip post home birth. But due to the disrespectful ways in which she was treated by an unkind male doctor, she quickly left the hospital without having allowed him to do even one single stitch:

> I, you know, I never got my vagina fixed. You know, so I had a year of where I couldn't have any sex or any pleasure because it was pretty, um—you know, I didn't really know what to make of it.

Venus needed a lot of time and effort to heal. Even still, during our interview, she'd told me that her sense of her sexual physiology had been changed, and had somehow been deepened by having given birth, which had continued throughout her healing journey from her first delivery:

> That outer labia on top of the hood of the clitoris was like totally ripped, you know? And so, I had a lot of scary feelings about that being pregnant again, and what would happen with the [second] birth, especially because I never got it fixed. But the midwives were aware of it ... I had to like, re-learn my body. But the amazing thing was that I started having vaginal orgasms after my first birth, because of the injury near my clitoris. So, it actually was a, you know—it paved this gateway that seemed like it—I don't know if it cleared out trauma or what but it—something about giving birth vaginally really like opened up my inner vaginal experience: my cervix and my uterus and my vaginal walls to more pleasure. So, I started having these deeper, deeper orgasms that weren't clitoral. So that was, you know, kind of neat.

In a sense, the attentiveness that Venus had needed to navigate this injury had led to an increased degree of awareness and sensitivity in areas that had previously been less involved in her sexual response process:

> When we did start making love again, because I was always avoiding that tear, or that place, I learned how to slow down and feel my insides more and like, move around the lingum [penis] in different ways. So, through that exploration, I learned a lot more about like, more circular sexuality and then actually feeling like the cavernous volume inside of my Yoni [vagina]. Like that there were all of these angles and things that I had never really been in touch with before. It feels like the baby passing through, like, awakens all of these little crevices. And so, from that, I was able to kind of stay with those sensations ... I got to explore all of that and just a way that I hadn't really known before. And then I naturally kind of began having orgasms that were not dependent on

> the clitoral orgasm. So that was good. And then it even felt better after the second baby … There was more connection with my breasts and just my whole body … you know, a lot more comfort with myself. But something physically changed. Definitely … I've had an incredible sex life after childbirth.

Aleks, after having given birth to four babies, two of which had been vaginal deliveries, had sensed a need for pelvic floor healing, and has adjusted their sex life accordingly:

> I needed to heal more this time around, you know. Four babies is not a joke. So, I actually, I still have a referral to a pelvic floor specialist, but then the pandemic or whatever. I think that I need to put it all back together again. I'm thinking of getting a peri-fit, which is this thing you put up there and then you play games on your phone, and you squeeze and get your muscles back on track. So, we haven't had as rough of sex as we do ordinarily. Because I'm not prepared yet for any of that kind of fisting and rough stuff, because I don't, I don't think it has fully healed. So, my previous labors taught me, you know, to be mindful of my body and the postpartum period. And that's what I'm doing right now.

Neutral or Mixed Impacts

Many of my study participants had not reported having experienced major changes in their sex lives postpartum, and so, I have little material to present within this theme. However, Melissa had indeed elaborated on how the relationship between birth and her sex life postpartum had been much more complex. Some aspects of her postpartum life had made having a satisfying sex life much more difficult; for example, her weight gain had negatively affected her sense of sexiness. Other positive changes had made having sex much better both for her and for her partner, such as her nipples having much more sensitivity.

> I breastfed my son for a year. Nipples are very sensitive, like much more sensitive than they were before I got pregnant. So that—it's like a new toy, I guess, inside some other pleasure point. But I mean, I am needing—I'm like 10 pounds heavier than I was before I had my son, which makes me less inclined to wear cute things. Maybe my husband misses that? I didn't even think about that. Um, but other than that, it's like the actual act is pretty much the same.

So, Melissa had not experienced the kinds of physical changes that Venus and Pearl discussed. She'd felt more or less unchanged by her birthing process, which also defies the general sociocultural narratives around the impacts of birth on the birthing body as being negative by default.

Negative Impacts

Some participants experienced negative changes to their sex lives postpartum. During our interview, Veronica, who is a practicing midwife, shared with me that she'd experienced what she'd been told was a minor tear at delivery, but that minor tear had turned out to be a major problem for both her sex life and her marriage.

> After the first baby, something bad happened to my perineum. Like, I don't know what it was because the midwife was like "You barely tore, you just had this one little—" like she did like a figure-eight stitch to repair it. So, she told me it was superficial, it didn't go into the muscles. But after that birth, depending on the angle of penetration, sometimes I get this horrible stinging and pulling sensation. And it was super uncomfortable. And I tried to get him to shift like angles. Then he'd get mad at me and say I was being bossy. And somehow, he's never gotten the message that I was trying to get him to not hurt me. And so, we'd get in fights about it … But maybe I never told him like "It hurts" because I thought it would hurt his feelings. And then the other thing is, when you're breastfeeding for a long time, you're in this very low estrogen state. So, your vaginal tissue kind of atrophies. I go back to my one year annual, and the midwife did an exam, and I was like, "That really hurts." So, she gave me vaginal estrogen cream, and it made a huge difference. But nobody told me that could happen. So, one thing I always tell breastfeeding moms, "If intercourse becomes uncomfortable in any way, shape, or form, stop. Come back right away, and we'll figure out why it hurts and then we'll fix it. Because if you have painful intercourse, it's going to ruin not just your sex life, but your relationship with your partner." That's some wisdom that came out of my own experience of not having that dealt with in a timely manner. And I mean, maybe it's part of why we have a bad relationship to this day. You know, that made a lot of problems in our relationship. But, I mean, if having sex always hurts, and then it feels like somebody like rubbed your vagina with sandpaper for four hours afterwards, it's sort of a buzzkill! [Laughs]

Callisto had a decrease in sexual desire after having her first baby. She attributed that change to her hormone levels and lamented not having been able to "get back" to her previous state of desire.

> I think I'm of the, you know, majority of women who have a decreased libido after having a baby. And, you know, I feel like hormonally, I haven't really been able to get back to where I was pre-birth. Just even like my sense of arousal, I feel like is different. Like, I don't have the same—it's not as easy for me to be aroused as it used to be like when I was like, 18, [laughs] ... much younger and childless.

Callisto had not experienced any positive changes in her sexual physiology postpartum either: "I wouldn't say it's gotten better and hasn't really gotten worse. So, I guess it's been about the same." Based on these interviews, I can say that the terrain in terms of sexual physicality postpartum seems to be quite varied. Still, the general cultural narratives weigh heavily on the negative while my data highlight a good deal of positive impacts of birth, particularly pleasurable birth, on birthing people's sexuality going forward.

Relational Factors

In our in-depth interviews, many participants talked about their sexuality in the context of their intimate relationships. Above I have presented some of my thematic findings concerning personal empowerment as well as the physiological changes participants experienced. Now I turn to the relational aspects, specifically the interpersonal issues that arose for the birthing person in ways that impacted their sexual lives, for better or worse, going forward. Some participants had seen improvements in their sexual relationships after birth. For others, birth pleasure experiences had not been linked to their sexual relationships at all. And still others had reported a diminished satisfaction with their sexual relationships postpartum. I start with those who reported no impact or a negative impact of birth on their sexual relationships. Then I will focus on those who reported that their birth pleasure experiences were beneficial to their sexual relationships.

Neutral and Negative Impacts

Several interview participants reported that their births had negative impacts on their sexual relationships. Veronica had a fraught relationship with her husband before their first birth, but her birth pleasure experience had not helped with that at all. If anything, in her mind, it had further alienated him from her, both physically and mentally because he'd played no meaningful role during the birth process. They'd been struggling through postpartum issues such as postpartum depression, sleep deprivation, and occupational stressors as well. During our interview, Veronica had explained:

> I'm kind of like, "How did I even get pregnant?" Because we had the older one in bed with us. And we were not getting along very well. And like he was trying to finish his dissertation, and I was—I had, like, horrendous postpartum depression where I was having like passive suicidal ideation on the daily. Like, I'd ride my bike to work and just think, "So I don't exactly want to die. But if I could just get hit by a bus and be laid up in traction on the top floor of the hospital for like three months, that sounds really, really nice." ... At some point, he told me this many, many years later. He was like, "Yeah, I got really mad at you and I decided we weren't going to have sex for a year." And so, for a year, apparently, we didn't have sex, but I didn't notice.

Even in situations without postpartum depression or any major stressors, sexual satisfaction is hard to come by for many postpartum people. Romi had also struggled with her sexual relationship with her husband, mostly in relational ways.

> We have a horrible sex life, I think. We've really struggled to find time. It's more about a time issue. So, my husband works late. And I'm a morning person, and he's a night owl. And so, it's been like—it just it doesn't work. And like, I'm not in my 20s I don't want to quickie in the closet, you know? Like, it's—we need it. We don't go to bed at the same time. And then my toddler just started sleeping in our bed. So, we've really struggled actually to find time to have sex. I know some couples are better at it. Also, like I'm a more sexual person than my husband is. And so, we've struggled in our relationship with just like, with, like, how to make that work. And we're kind of talking about it again, we're trying to figure out how to make it work. And it's been, it's like—I love my husband; we have such a strong relationship. But it's an area of disconnect, where we're going to continue to struggle with this throughout our lives. So unfortunately, it hasn't improved.

During our interview, Fabia too had shared a general understanding of universal difficulty in this regard:

> When you have the little one it's just so, so difficult. And you're so tired that to have sex is just like very, very difficult. Yeah, my sex life after like

> within the first couple of years—I can't remember any of it. So, I guess there wasn't a lot of it.

Fabia had also found that breastfeeding eliminated her libido. Sex during that breastfeeding phase had been described by several study participants as having been a sacrifice for the sake of the partner. In Fabia's words: "I think my sex life was more about [my husband] than it was about me because I was nursing and I just my libido was just like … 'Now's not the time for you to get pregnant. You have to look after this little one.' "

Eventually, Fabia's sexual relationship with her husband improved, but she had not credited her pleasurable birthing experience for this in any way. In her words:

> Sex has definitely gotten much, much better. But I think it's just because we've been longer together. And we love each other very much … I'm not—I wouldn't—I don't think having a child has made a difference. I think it's that we've been together longer is what has made the difference.

Malika had relational issues with her partner lingering since the pregnancy, when she'd had spikes in her sexual desire and her partner had refused all sexual contact out of unnecessary fear of hurting the baby during sex. As she explained:

> There were a time a couple of times in my pregnancy when I really did feel like super sexual, like I really wanted to have sex. But at the time … —my fiancé—felt like he was gonna hurt the baby. He didn't want to have sex. To this day, I'm still kind of annoyed by it because I felt like he wasn't really being attentive to me.

Postpartum, there'd been physical sexual issues with her partner's body that had continued to interrupt their worsening sexual relationship.

> He had something that happened to him. I think it's called priapism where he had to, he had to have surgery on his penis because he had an erection that lasted over 24 hours. So, my daughter is actually a miracle baby. But ever since—ever since I healed after having her, we still haven't had sex yet. Because his penis is still not quite working the way it's supposed to.

These complexities, when added to the mix of postpartum pressures, had created both a tense and disappointing sexual reality for Malika, and, during our interview, she'd shared with me her desire to improve her sex life. Araceli too had heightened sexual needs during pregnancy that impacted their sexual relationship.

> I think it was definitely sexual during my first pregnancy. Because there was no fear. Maybe there's some, you know, part of the thing I haven't mentioned is I had two miscarriages before [firstborn]. And so, there was a little bit of fear that like this pregnancy wasn't gonna work out either. So, like the first three months, were just like, "We're not doing anything to endanger the situation." But I think we definitely had sex, and just not a lot. It was kind of fun. It was fun to have sex while pregnant.

But Araceli, in the aftermath of the traumatic birth she experienced, felt betrayed by her partner and lost all sexual interest in him:

> Having the child definitely changed the relationship. And then there was like, zero sex after that, like, we just like—I could not abide. "No Entry." Also, like, and socio-emotionally I felt betrayed, or I don't know, like, of course, part of the trauma was like, you know, "I trusted you, but I don't think I can trust you because you didn't know what to do. Like, even though we tried really hard at knowing what to do. You didn't know how to help me." Of course, I didn't know how to help myself. But anyway, so there was a lot of betrayal sort of there. And so, then we just like had a broken relationship. And when we made up once we got pregnant with [our second born] ... But then there was no more sex ever again. Basically, since [the second born]. I have my own devices to have—I have my own pleasure and release whenever it is needed. But uh, yeah, we haven't had sex since ... I don't long for that intimacy. I feel like nursing for four years is definitely a turnoff for intimacy. Because you're over-touched and sassy.

And so, multiple factors had entwined during our interview: her previous birth traumas and breastfeeding had combined to eliminate Araceli's sexual relationship with her husband. Melissa also had experienced a complex relationship with her sexuality throughout her pregnancy, when her sexual relationship with her husband had taken on an obligatory cast:

> I'm a very sexual person. Love to have sex. But from the moment I started to feel my baby, like real hard kicks during pregnancy, it'd be so hard for me to have sex and be completely into that. And like feeling the baby move at the same time, it was just trippy in my mind, and after a while,

> I was like, “No, like, we can’t do this anymore.” Because I was too much in my head. And you know, just being bigger and uncomfortable. So, during sex, I’d say like, after my—sixth [month]? I guess we had sex until like the eighth month, but it was truly me just trying to be a good wife. Taking one for the team.

When the birth of the baby finally came, Melissa was thrilled to get back to her vibrant, enthusiastic sexual relationship with her husband, in spite of the postpartum challenges they faced:

> After [birth] I was like, I missed it [sex] so much, because we hadn’t had sex towards the end of my pregnancy, that I just—I wanted it [Laughs] so bad. Um, and yeah, we were a relatively young couple. We got married in September, and I found out I was pregnant in November. So, we were just like, still at the height of our honeymoon phase. And then it got put on pause for pregnancy. So, we were happy to jump right back into it. And it’s been, I mean, when you have a newborn you’re tired a lot, you know, don’t have time, but we figured out like ways to make it work. And now that my son is more in a routine it’s really back to normal. And then thinking about having another baby, I’m like “Do I really—?” I don’t want to give up this whole free sex [laughs] for a newborn life! But I’ll take one for the team? I’m good at that. I’m good at [Laughs], at taking one for the team. Yeah, um, sex is—sex is amazing!

In Melissa’s case, having sex had returned her to a highly satisfying and to a normal postpartum period, with some work. During our interview, Aleks had also told me all about the complexities, the difficulties, the lack of privacy, and the fatigue of raising children and keeping their sexual life thriving:

> So, we first of all, we don’t have the time. Second of all, we have four kids. And we don’t want them to hear. My mom comes, rarely. So, sex has been few and far between. And someone has to be here to like, watch all the other kids and we have to lock the door. So, it’s really different.

Beyond these issues, however, Aleks had postulated that their wife’s view of their birthing body as sexy, capable, and exciting had probably been greatly enhanced by their having witnessed the birth of their child:

> I think it was something for her [my wife] to see me do this [give birth]. That that reinforced in her mind, like, what a badass I am and how she finds that really sexy. I think she’d tell you that. That watching me through labor was like an experience, [laughs] a pleasurable experience.

This sentiment about shifts in how the partner feels about the birthing person came up in my interviews with Sankofa and Skylar as well. This relational element, which is a recognition of power and a sense of awe in response to witnessing birth, is counter to the standard, often sexist sociocultural narratives about the birthing body being "repulsive," "scary," "too much," and generally "gross," in particular for male partners of birthing people. So, partners, men in particular, who'd been highly involved and excited to participate in the birthing process defy those extremely negative and insulting narratives.

To summarize, there are many dynamics within pregnancy, birth, and the postpartum period that interrupt sexual relationality or threaten to destroy it altogether. Physical changes, new pressures, stressors, trauma, and spatial constraints had heavily impinged on these participants' sexual relationships. These factors had conspired in ways that had greatly reduced sexual satisfaction for many of these participants. Now, I will focus on positive relational impacts following pleasurable birth experiences.

Positive Impacts

Several study participants had reported deeper and much more satisfying sexual relationships with their partners as the result of having together experienced pregnancy and birth. During our interview, Sankofa is one who'd highlighted the ways in which the intimacy between her husband and her had greatly deepened over the course of her four births, and how she now practices sexual connection with her husband and shares those practices with others:

> I tell people like really looking in your partner's eyes when you're making love, letting your third eyes connect, feeling each other's heartbeat … really breathing—breath work—and all those things, kind of leading up to the actual event can be very, very, just connecting and grounding for a couple. So, for me, it's been so much better because I have more of an understanding of my own body. I feel like he has more respect for my body witnessing me give birth several times. So yeah, it's been better for us.

Sankofa had, however, acknowledged the reality for many others who feel that the fire of their sexual relationship has died down, and yet, from an obligatory place, tolerate unwanted sex:

> But I've heard some stories where some of my friends are like "Oh, I just do it to tolerate it." And I'm like, "Oh, that makes me feel so sad." You know that [laughs], because I can't imagine having that disconnect and

> then feeling obligated to kind of fulfill somebody else's needs, but not really like whole-heartedly to want to be there.

Marion had fully fit into this same description early in her marriage, when sexual difficulties were compounded by the trauma she experienced in her first birth. But she credited her powerful second birth experience with her growth into a new, freer, more expressive kind of sexual relationship with her husband:

> My husband was my first sexual experience. I was raised Christian, and we waited and all that. And it was lovely, but I didn't have a very satisfying sexual relationship with him because immediately we got pregnant. And pregnancy hormones and me and sex, like, don't work out. I get heartburn. There's no having an orgasm when I'm pregnant. It just hurts. And so, I went through the first pregnancy, then postpartum depression.

For Marion, the relationality of her second birth had been a notable aspect of the pleasure that she'd experienced, and she'd connected this relationality to their much deeper sexual connection and to their heightened sexual satisfaction:

> My birth was like, the best day of my life! And it was probably better than most of my sexual experiences, like just in the, the holistic aspect of everything being so beautiful and perfect, and bonding between me my husband, myself, and me, and this little one, like that's, that's pleasurable, too.

Marion had continued by saying that it had been during her second pregnancy that pleasure during sex had experientially started to happen for her:

> I didn't really learn how to experience pleasure. And he hadn't really learned what I needed until pretty close to [baby]'s birth, or the middle of the [second] pregnancy … And I was like, "Alright, now things are getting good! That's fun!" Um, but as soon as [baby] was out, I was like, "Whoa! I am powerful. I have no belly in the way! I'm going to do whatever I want!" … And ah, wow. So much better. Like, so satisfying, and so much more fun! [laughs]. Yeah, it's, it's been a journey for us to kind of get there and figure it out.

Skylar had also matched this obligatory dynamic during the early days of her marriage: "Initially, it had been like, once a week, and just was—it was more like a chore versus, you know, a pleasurable time." Their sexual relationship had deepened considerably after her second birth, but it was something that she had not thought much about until our interview:

> We really grew very close after that [second birth]. Um, and, um ... yeah. I guess I never really thought much about it all. For a while, until probably when my son [second born] was three months old, I thought about it more. And I was like, "Oh!" You know? Things improved significantly! [laughs]

Skylar had attributed part of this significant development to the healing work that she'd already done on herself, and, during our interview, noted that this most fortunate development has resulted in a much more satisfying relationship with her husband:

> After my daughter was born [first birth], I was taking the time to build my self-confidence, build my self-image, and just kind of focus on me a little bit more. And I think in the result of me doing that, as well, and then continuing to do it after my son was born, that played a huge, huge, huge role in my husband and I's sex life. Because I didn't have great experiences with boyfriends prior to my husband. And those really kind of tore me up in a lot of ways. And so then—I kind of lost who I was. And then through the process of having both of my kids and then growing as much as I have, I got that confidence back. And I reopened to my husband in a way that I'd never opened up to him.

Bree had also fit into this pattern of a previous approach to a sexual relationship that had deprioritized herself and had primarily been "for him." In her words:

> I mean, obviously, my husband and I don't have as much sex as we used to. And I think it's really just because I'm tired [Laughs]. Having a child is really, really hard. And it's been a balance to take care of her as well as myself, and then also give attention to my husband. So, we don't have sex as much as I'd like to. But when we do, it's a really profound connection that we have. Because I experience my body in such a different way that now, when I share it with him, it's completely different ... I'm just more comfortable with telling him what I want. I'm not afraid to direct him and basically tell him how I like to be pleasured. Because before it felt like I was having sex *for* him. Like, it was never

> about me. And now it's a lot more about me, but I mean, both of us, but I'm including myself a lot more in the process.

Bree was "thrilled" to share during our interview that her sexual relationship had become vastly more satisfying having gone through birth and the personal transformation and empowerment that it provided to her:

> [Sex is] a lot better, because now, you know—obviously, people can't read your mind. So, you have to tell them and not obviously, like, in a forceful or like dictating way, but I try to be very conscious of the way I—how, like how I direct him. But it's a lot better, because now I'm actually not sitting there, laying there, like thinking like, "I wish he would do this." It's a lot more enjoyable for me now, because I'm enjoying myself. Now I'm not sitting around waiting and hoping that he's gonna do what I want him to. But he doesn't know what I'm thinking unless I say something. So, I've really learned to communicate a lot better. And in turn, I'm getting what I want. And then he's also getting what he wants. Because obviously, you know, he finds pleasure in pleasuring me and vice versa. So, we have a really symbiotic relationship now when it comes to that. Because before it was a little—it was very one-sided. And I was always left, kind of—not resenting him, but not feeling fully satisfied.

Nava had also reported a positive shift in relationality between her and her partner during the immediate afterglow of their first birth:

> I started feeling better [postpartum]. I noticed a kind of really really strong, like, chemistry between me and [my partner] and I felt wasn't there since the beginning of our relationship. Like that really strong spark that brought us together. I felt all of a sudden it sort of came back. And I was surprised because I expected you know, sleep deprivation, and with the baby, and like all that, that it just wouldn't—that it would kind of go away for a while. I felt like, I don't know, it was really crazy. We haven't had sex yet since because I'm waiting to fully heal. But—I think—I don't know, something has changed for us in a very positive way since. And I don't know if I can necessarily attribute that—But I think we don't take each other for granted as much now, because we don't have that intimate time as available, as accessible. So, it's, um, that might be part of it. Or maybe some hormonal changes too. I'm not sure. But it's been really refreshing. And really good for us that we have this like this new, strong—not new but kind of refreshed, rejuvenated passion for one another.

For all of these study participants, the shifts in their self-images that had occurred during their pleasurable births had eventually carried over to their sexual relationships, and they'd gained much deeper senses of their sexual bodily autonomies, their closeness to and their openness with their partners. These factors had allowed for more satisfying sexual relationships even in the new complexities that come with the newborn phase. With a new sense of self-regard after birth, these participants were better able to own their sexual desires, to share them with their partners in new ways, and in return, to gain much more satisfaction from their sexual relationships. This thematic finding runs counter to the standard and negative sociocultural narratives of postpartum sexuality and demonstrates the wide variability in the ways birth is experienced, and the impacts that birth can have on birthing people's sexual lives going forward.

Gender and Sexual Orientation

Themes related to gender and sexual orientation emerged in the interviews in a myriad of ways. Some participants dealt with both sexist and cisheteronormative oppressions. There'd also been pleasure associated with gender affirmation for the ciswomen as well as, in a more nuanced way, for the agender and nonbinary participants whom I'd interviewed. Sexual orientation had also involved a paradoxical range of both oppressive and liberatory energies during birth, particularly for those who'd given birth in their own homes and thus, had more latitude for relational or even sexual expression. First, I present the emergent themes on gender, and then on sexual orientation, as they'd related to the multiple types of pleasure experienced in the birth process (affirmatively or antagonistically).

Gender

During our interviews, gender had emerged as an important theme in three main ways. First, sexism and misogyny had been experienced in many ways throughout the participants' reproductive lives, particularly at the moment of birth for those who'd experienced obstetric violence or traumatic births. Debbie, in particular, had identified both the sexism and the misogyny that had explicitly been the root causes of the obstetric violence that she'd endured in the hospital during her first birth, specifically the demeaning treatment she endured and also the harmful "Daddy Stitches." "Daddy Stitches" are unnecessary vaginal sutures performed post-birth that make the vaginal opening much smaller as they heal. As the name implies, these are performed, often with a wink, for the presumed sexual gratification of male sexual partners. Aleks, who self-identified as an agender lesbian, had also seen their bodily experiences of birth within the context of sexist oppression as a feminist statement:

> It was like finally understanding that it [birth] is not a personal journey, and yet you can be a person who resists institutions. And seeing my [own] mother, finally, as part of these institutions as well—not that I forgive a lot of it, but I can feel better understanding her existence as well, and her experiences. And how much of it comes down to bodily autonomy, and that being political. And both something you process intimately with people sometimes or privately within yourself. But also, in making decisions about your body, you're making a political feminist statement.

Most participants, regardless of their gender identities, had fully identified with feminist ideas such as valuing gender equality between men and women/femmes, and gender expansive people. But some had eschewed the label "feminist" for various reasons (typically conservative cisgender women).

Second, gender expression was associated to birth with its own kinds of pleasure. I call these kinds of pleasure "gender pleasure," and define them as: "pleasure that has been derived from feeling an embodied alignment with one's own gender identity." In some ways, it might be thought of as the opposite of gender dysphoria, which is defined in the DSM-5 (the Diagnostic and Statistical Manual of Mental Disorders, 5th edition) (American Psychiatric Association, 2022) as a "marked incongruence between an individual's gender identity and assigned gender, with associated distress or impairment" (Cooper et al., 2020). For some ciswomen interview participants, this gender pleasure involved archetypal cultural imagery, such as identifying as a mother, a goddess, or a feminine divine being. For example, during our interview, Venus shared: "I felt so powerful! And again, just that. It's like this euphoric power. Yeah, I felt like the goddess herself!" These kinds of imagery had sometimes been expressed as having been "spiritual pleasures," manifest as a deep sense of connection with their lineage of mothers, of mothers all over the world, in an expansive, spiritual way. For example, Romi had felt that her pleasurable birth experience had connected her to other women in a deeper way:

> It was almost like a spiritual and religious experience, like accessing this other part of the human experience, the female experience, and which is obviously tremendously powerful and sort of connects you to your history and all the women in the world. And it's just, it's powerful. I'm like, I'm getting emotional as I talk about it.

For gender nonbinary or agender folks, "gender pleasure" involved fully embodying their own unique relationship to their gender whist giving birth, beyond or despite the constraints of the cisheteronormativity of typical maternal care and of "motherhood" as a femme gendered societal and/or cultural construction.

Third, gender had also been discussed in terms of matrescence (Davis-Floyd, 2022; Orchard et al., 2023) or as a sense of moving through a rite of passage as a woman in the birth experience (see Davis-Floyd, 2022), and that this transformation from non-motherhood to motherhood (and/or from non-parenthood to parenthood) had engendered certain kinds of pleasure, a deeper sense of self-awareness and self-love, and a new sense of one's gender identity. During our interview, Araceli had shared with me a bit about how her eyes had been opened and her sense of her own identity had shifted as she moved through the embodied stages of reproduction and their associated realms of experiential knowledge, which she called "clubs" that had re-shaped her sense of her gendered self in the world at large:

> When I finally decided that I wanted to have children, it was like "This is a different experience in the world." Like going through birth is something that I wanted to live through. I wanted to live through that. Birth—like pregnancy—birthing. I want to live through that—I need to understand this to be a full-fledged woman—human. And of course, parenthood, I really had no idea. Like it's just—like we can't know until we do it. There's just no way of knowing it. How it is all-encompassing? Right? And so yeah, like I probably walk around the world as a parent now, and parents are not the same as whatever single non-parent people. So, there's like multiple clubs that this progression has meant. It was like the "Pregnancy Club." That's one. [laughs] There's the "Birth Club." That's another one. There's like the "Natural Birth Club." That's another one. And the like "Motherhood" is another one. And "Motherhood plus being single breadwinner in a home" is also another one, right? Like there's just "Working Mother." And it does make me advocate more for the people who I feel like, "Holy cow! There's this whole other set of needs that people like me have or don't have, or don't get addressed, right? Their needs don't get addressed.

Building on that sentiment, Venus had articulated a reclamation of mothering in a feminist sense, in defiance of a belittled stereotype, a stereotype that she'd admittedly bought into for much of her adulthood:

> I feel more of that just responsibility for mothering others. I have a lot of young women who I mentor, you know? And I think that all that

> has come from really embracing the, the power of the Divine Mother, who I think has been missing for a while, and—feminism is awesome. And it's been so important, but some of the initial backlash was some hardness. And so, I—you know, I feel like I'm able to really embrace the good qualities of mothering, you know, and not—and not—and not be—not feel like I'm torn down by it. Like, it's okay that I am one of those moms who cooks for everyone. You know? ... It's just, it's just a reclaiming of these feminine things that I think are really important to keep the thread of society together.

Agender and nonbinary birth parents Aleks and Cande spoke at length about gender and about the ways their gender expressions were protected within their chosen birth spaces, and with their chosen support teams. Cande had navigated their pregnancy and birth during the COVID-19 lockdown, and, during our interview, had explained to me about how their gender identity experience had been nuanced throughout the process, and had, in some ways, been shielded from the expected public scrutiny that gender-expansive people often face:

> I identify as non-binary queer. And so, I definitely identify as the mother, or I mean, not as a mother—as a parent. So having a lot of navigating of like, like, "Oh, Mommy!" and I'm like, "No, I'm Maddy" [a gender-expansive term for a parent]. And they're like, "What?" But yes, like, identifying—the transition to parent has been interesting ... I guess, mostly because I didn't know if it would ever happen. I wasn't one of those people that like, nursed dolls when they were a kid, or like, had these like huge, innate internal desires of like, being a parent. Not that there's anything wrong with those that do. But it just wasn't my route. And I think my identity as a parent also is very much intertwined with COVID. And the fact that like, I don't go anywhere, I don't see anybody. And though I haven't really had to navigate a lot of like overly patriarchal assumed gender stereotypes ... [and] the public scrutiny of identifying as non-binary, which I think in one regard, I'm very lucky for that. I also found that being pregnant affected my own identity, and like, I embraced more of my internal femininity when I was pregnant. And now I'm—not that I'm against any of it—I just, it's just, I don't know. I've always believed that [gender] is a very fluid thing. But assumptions of like parenthood is—there's all these like, assumptions of like, "Okay, well, you're a mother?" ... And I'm just kind of like, "Eh eh eh." I'm gonna feed the kid because I can, in the ways in which I want to. But like, I don't know, I don't know if I like—I mean, I obviously identify as a parent, because I have kids now. I shouldn't say obviously. Just

> because you have a kid doesn't mean you identify as a parent. But it's sort of been cocooned within the house that I live in with my partner. And so, it's sometimes weird.

A "cocoon of safety" had also been an important theme during Aleks's interview. Throughout Aleks's home birth, they'd felt lovingly held within their own space, surrounded by queer women and queer people. Aleks had firmly rebuked any femme imaginary of the divine feminine as was mentioned by several ciswomen participants. Aleks had specifically linked their birthing pleasure to the pursuit of those "unapologetic" queer spaces, and to the kind of labor that had been required to create these spaces:

> It's really something to have people try to find some joy and build their families against all odds—when the country and the laws are trying to say you're not worthy of having a baby ... How can you find pleasure and joy in all this fear and lack of support? And how do you do it? Like, who do you find to support you?

Aleks had also envisioned developing scholarly research on the processes of creating loving spaces of care for the reproductive dreams of gender expansive people:

> I think it is much more complicated to the person that I am now because I'm much more complicated as a person. And so, it's now going to take these embodied conversations for trans and non-binary people about how they make decisions about fertility and face infertility. And it's going to be like a mixture of talking about forging paths when there are no models for it. And these people, we, I mean, I'm these people, we are making our own paths with—with—despite what everybody says. But also getting at the lack of institutional access and care and the way healthcare settings are deeply abusive to transgender and non-binary people, especially during pregnancy and labor. And, and so it's, it's gonna bring together this like, deep personal embodiment, and, and structural inequality that I find that I can finally now conceptualize in this person that I am.

Aleks had said so much during our interview that it could warrant its own chapter. But suffice it to say, for the sake of the scope of this book, that birth pleasure and queer birth are both rebellions. Being guided by pleasure into one's birthing process is non-normative; it defies the typical individual, social, and cultural mindsets about birth and family-building. Gender-expansive people experience the impacts of these cisheteronormative mindsets on many levels, both internally and externally. And the paths that they are presently forging, "against all odds," as Aleks had quite aptly put it, into parenthood, are beset on all sides by escalating sociocultural opposition, cisheteronormativity, and sexual oppression. Experiencing pleasure in the face of all this antagonism is its own kind of defiance.

Sexual Orientation

Four of the 23 study participants identified as lesbian and/or queer. Two participants identified as bisexual, and two more as "mostly heterosexual." The remaining 15 identified as straight or heterosexual. Sexual orientation had not been a major theme in most interviews, across sexual orientations. Those who identified as bisexual at the time of our interviews had been in long-term committed relationships (specifically marriage, non-polyamorous at the time) with men. Their sexual orientations had not emerged in our interviews as a major aspect of their birth experiences either. The same can be said for those who identified as mostly heterosexual, and those who identified as exclusively heterosexual. Those who identified as queer and/or lesbian at the time of our interviews had varied in the salience of their sexual orientation to the various types of pleasure that they'd experienced during their births. But of any group, this group had the most to say about their sexual orientations; thus, I expand on their experiences next.

The four interview participants who identified as queer and/or lesbian included Aleks, Cande, Semiramis, and Theia. The ways in which their sexual orientations had factored into their birth pleasure experiences had not been uniform. First, although Theia and Semiramis identified as queer/lesbians at the time of our interviews, their descriptions of their pleasurable birth experiences had not included any references to their sexual orientations, and at the times of their births, they'd both been in heterosexual relationships with men. Cande also identified as queer, but this identity was not highlighted as they described their birth experience in the autonomous birth center. During our interview, Cande had shared with me that they'd self-stimulated sexual pleasure while they'd been in labor at home, and reported that method contrasted with the intensity of their contractions, and that they'd experienced orgasms as a result of this self-stimulation. But they had not described the practice of self-stimulation in a way that had drawn in their sexual identity or sexual orientation. In their words:

> I actually had orgasms while I was like—as a way to counteract the contractions ... Self-stimulation as a way to sort of counteract the

> contractions … through like labor, there were orgasms, which, I guess is a huge thing about pleasure.

Little more was shared about this orgasmic aspect of their experience. Aleks, however, had drawn deep connections between their sexual orientation and their also pleasurable birth experiences. From the very start of their labor during their most recent home birth, multiple types of pleasure had been salient to them. In their own words:

> I remember thinking that I want to wear something that feels good to my body, that I look good in or something that my wife likes. And so, there's this shirt that I wore that she likes that I like, and how it feels. So, it immediately became something connected to sensation and pleasure. I was just like "How do I want to feel?" And through this labor and before the doula got there were like a lot of intimate moments with my wife.

For Aleks, their sexual orientation had been woven into their relatedness with their entire birth care team, including their wife and the queer women and people whom they'd chosen to be there for their home birth. Although I have quoted this interview above regarding sexual pleasure during birth, here I include it once more to emphasize how sexual orientation can be integral to the birth experience:

> I just allowed myself to be very primal—animalistic, and like, move with the labor instead of like worrying how I'm seen. But there was really something to having queer women and queer people around me. I had a queer friend come over as well, with whom like we have flirtatious friendships and, and there's also something to the doula being queer. Like, I was naked in front of these women. And there is a pleasure to that. And not only was I naked in front of these women, and we were all queer, but I was like, able to be just open, right? And like, peeing and bleeding, and pooping. I had a bucket. [laughs] I was joking around with them. And then I was like bearing into the bucket, and all of these things were coming out. And every once in a while, my wife would empty it—and I just thought, "What an incredible experience!" It was like embodied and flirtatious and sexual, and they were joking about other things and like, just talking to each other, and I just was like—first of all, I find all of these people attractive simultaneously. Second of all, I'm like, in love with what's taking place right now, because labor takes time. It's a process. And so, while I crouch down, and I do all of

> this, and I would use the staircase for support, and I would open into a crouch low on the floor, you know? I just was thinking how much this feels like the sex parties that we attend, to some extent with people around, kind of moving around and doing their own thing, but you're also doing something with your body, but like, times 1000, because there's a baby coming, you know? So, it was a very queer experience, very sexual in that way.

In these ways, for Aleks, the various types of pleasure they'd experienced and their sexual orientation were deeply entwined. The birth space, the physicality, and the relationality all fully resonated with their gender and sexual identity in a way that had given them pleasure and had not disrupted their birthing process but rather had fully supported its unfolding. Thematically, the birthing experiences that I've documented herein align with the themes that I've described in the previous sections of this chapter that have dealt with the contexts wherein many types of pleasure can occur. Safety, privacy, freedom of self-expression, deep connections with others, and full bodily autonomy echoed throughout Aleks's interview and so many others as the fundamental bedrocks of pleasure in the birth process.

References

American Psychiatric Association. (2022). *Diagnostic and statistical manual of mental disorders* (5th ed., text rev.). https://doi.org/10.1176/appi.books.9780890425787

Cooper, K., Russell, A., Mandy, W., & Butler, C. (2020). The phenomenology of gender dysphoria in adults: A systematic review and meta-synthesis. *Clinical Psychology Review*, *80*, 101875. https://doi.org/10.1016/j.cpr.2020.10187

Davis-Floyd, R. (2022). *Birth as an American rite of passage* (3rd ed.). Routledge.

Orchard, E. R., Rutherford, H. J., Holmes, A. J., & Jamadar, S. D. (2023). Matrescence: Lifetime impact of motherhood on cognition and the brain. *Trends in Cognitive Sciences*. https://doi.org/10.1016/j.tics.2022.12.002

6

RACE, CLASS, AND FEELING GOOD IN BIRTH

> And I felt surges and surges and surges of, oh my God, it just felt *really good*. [Long pause]. People don't understand. [Laughs]. You know? *I just felt so good*, like incredible wellbeing. *Incredible wellbeing*.
>
> Chandra

If I could, I would have my readers start this chapter by listening to the unforgettable Nina Simone's song: "Feeling Good" (1965). In this song, this iconoclastic Black woman civil rights activist juxtaposes minimalist lyrics about life's simple, beautiful pleasures with menacing tones and a plodding tempo. She helps her listeners to understand that the experience of pleasure in the face of oppression is dangerously revolutionary. How else to better start this chapter?

In this section, I address the ways in which the important topics of both race and class emerged as both distinct and entangled in many of my interviews, specifically regarding how my study's participants had connected their experiences of pleasure during birth to their racial identities and class positionalities. I must note that I will use gender-appropriate language as determined by how interview participants had identified themselves, and so I use "women" and "mothers" and/or "parent(s)" or "birthing person(s)" to intentionally honor these self-designations. Herein, I group participants by race because race had most definitely been the most salient self-identification raised by racialized study participants during our interviews. Class, however, had emerged for many participants less as an identity and more as a way to speak with clarity as to how they'd navigated

DOI: 10.4324/9781003499428-7

their birth care: those who'd had financial privileges had cleverly leveraged them, those who had not enjoyed such privileges and had both faced and contested their financial barriers. By grouping participants on the basis of race, I have not intended to flatten their identities or experiences, but rather to provide a more focused way to interrogate how both race and racism had shown up during their labor and birth experiences and had intersected with their class positions. While reading this section, I advise my readers to refer to the chart in the Appendix to this book for further details and nuances on each unique and incredible study participant. I will also refer back to sections where specific birth experiences were covered in depth in preceding chapters. However, before I dive into these intersectional analyses in the following sections of this chapter, I briefly sketch out an overarching analysis of the class-related characteristics across all of my study participants.

Class

I recruited my study participants from across broad spectra of racial and class-based social positions (for details on the study design and participation breakdown, again, see the Appendix). Class is typically studied within the healthcare realm as "socioeconomic status," a social and structural determinant of health that is measured as a composite of income, education, and occupation (Crear-Perry et al., 2021; Easterbrook et al., 2020; Nam & Terrie, 2021). I chose to include housing status as another key salient category that had emerged during these interviews (Rolfe et al., 2020). There are many ways to measure these socioeconomic factors, but here, as a part of my qualitative study, I sought overarching themes which I present below by major category, as they'd been related to the many types of pleasure that can experienced during birth. (See Chapter 5.)

Income

Study participants had a wide range of annual incomes. At the time of our interviews, the mean family income was US$95,652 per year (range of $18,000–$300,000 per year, and the family size ranged from 2 to 7). Although I do not intend to provide a representative analysis of income and race, I do want to include how income looked across race. White participants had the lowest average annual income at $70,455, followed by mixed identity participants with $72,500, Black participants with $86,800, Latina/es with $98,000, and Asian/Pacific Islanders had the highest with $216,667 per year. When I'd included Semiramis (White and

MENA—Middle Eastern and North African) in the "White" category and Melissa in either the "Black" or the "Latina/e" categories, they'd raised the averages of each to $71,091 (White), $92,333 (Black), and $105,333 (Latina/es). Across the board during our interviews, money had been cited as a major factor for having access to quality personalized birth support such as a doula, a homebirth midwife, or superior medical health care through private health insurance as compared to public health insurance that is available only to those who fall below a quite low threshold, at least in the United States. The study participants who'd been living in the US at the time of our interviews, who'd had the funds to access care that aligned with their preferences recognized this ability as a privilege. The participants who'd been living outside of the US had different healthcare structures to contend with, but at least for one, Nava in Israel, the Israeli marginalization of midwifery from their coverage model of maternal care made home birth difficult to access for lower- or middle-income people. Fabia, from Spain but living in the United Kingdom at the time of our interview, gave birth at home unattended by any care providers ("free-birth"), and in this way had not engaged with the formal care system.

Education

I asked my study participants about the highest level of education that they had completed. One participant had completed high school only, four had completed some college or trade school, two had bachelor's degrees, and the 16 remaining participants had master's, professional, or doctoral degrees. Generally, the people whom I interviewed had invested time and energy into preparing themselves for birth through childbirth education of different kinds. Most participants cited their desire for full and nuanced information about birth, and their confidence in seeking out that information had been an important part of how they'd navigated their pregnancies. In that childbirth education process, some participants discovered the possibility that birth can be pleasurable or even pain-free.

Occupation

Work was addressed in most interviews. At the time of our interviews, some study participants had been stay-at-home parents or students with little to no income. Others were commanding high salaries in careers as researchers, consultants, tenure-track assistant professors, full professors, designers, therapists, and business owners. Many study participants had fully been engaged in birth work as doulas or midwives as their full-time or part-time profession. Some participants had worked until the day they went into labor, and others had taken time off long before their due dates. Some returned to work very soon after birth, and others never had because they'd decided to become stay-at-home mothers and/or parents. Intersecting sociocultural dynamics affected the working lives of these birthing people, and in turn their working lives affected their birth experiences. Additionally, this interplay between work and reproductive life was complicated and layered by issues such as financial need or relationship factors such as a sudden divorce. With all this diversity in occupational experience to attend to in this study, only a few themes have stood out overall. First and most salient is the connection of occupation to birth pleasure is stress. Stressors leading up to birth, particularly if the baby had been born earlier than expected, had required some amelioration for pleasure to be experienced. For working mothers or birth parents who had their babies earlier than expected, their preparation had been cut short—they'd not had the time that they'd anticipated to take childbirth preparation courses, for example, or to otherwise get themselves ready for birth. This lack of time had been an added stressor in an already stressful situation. On a different note, after having had such an incredible experience of birth, some study participants were inspired to go into birthwork as doulas or midwives.

Housing

Housing is without a doubt a class issue that affects birthing people's experiences of birth. Fundamentally, access to the full spectrum of birth care options, like home birth, is curtailed for someone who is unhoused. The quality and autonomy of one's living space impacts these choices as well. A sense of privacy is not universal, even in a dwelling that is one's own. Shared walls and dense spaces where sound travels can all impact the experiences of safety and privacy of an apartment, for example. Some participants had addressed housing as having been an important issue in their birth journeys, mostly emphasizing the pleasure of birthing in their own spaces, but also in the absence of steady housing, the impact of that absence on the birthing body. For example, Theia and Nava had been living with family members during their pregnancies, which had shaped their birth setting choices and their experiences of privacy, intimacy, and a sense of family participation in the birthing process. For privacy, Nava had chosen to give birth in an autonomous birth center, and her transport to this center had been the most painful and unpleasant part of her birthing experience. Theia had given birth in her own home, a unit downstairs from her parents. She'd been happy with the fact that her family members were right upstairs the whole time, close but not overly involved. Her older children participated in some of the most precious moments of her birthing process, a moving and a cherished experience for her. For another example, Malika and her family had been facing housing instability at the time of her birth and had been unhoused at the time of our interview. Her initial choice to give birth in an autonomous birth center had, in part, been motivated by her concern for her privacy.

All of these class-related aspects collide with racism. Poverty is racist. Educational attainment is besieged by racial inequities from top to bottom, as is the working world. Housing injustice is the product of well-documented racist land, housing, and financial policies in the US, such as red-lining (which is a range of racist practices that include, for example, systematic exclusion from the housing market by refusing to approve mortgages in "red-lined" neighborhoods, as well as other market-shaping designations that suppress the value of the housing stock in "red-lined" Black and Brown neighborhoods), and long-standing and genocidal policies of land theft, murder, and displacement of Indigenous peoples across the continent. I mention these not to be exhaustive, an impossible feat in this book, but to raise the reader's awareness of the interconnectedness of these oppressive legacies with current struggles for both reproductive and birth justice. I feel I must at minimum name these interacting dynamics, even while naming them is sorely insufficient.

Through critical feminist and intersectional lenses (Crenshaw, 1989), next I will focus in on the study participants' views on the ways in which race, racism, and class had come to bear on their pleasurable experiences of birth. I start by centering the five Black women with whom I conducted interviews—Chandra, Callie, Malika, Callisto, Sankofa, and, also Melissa, who identified as mixed-race Black and Latina. I then weave Melissa's births into the next section, which is focused on Latina/Latine/Latinx people, along with Araceli (Mexican-American binational) and Cande (Mexican Mestiza). Then I turn to the three Asian/Pacific Islander participants Bree (Vietnamese), Dalisay (Filipina), and Raquel (Chinese). Next, I address the participants who identified as White. I also present findings from those with Middle Eastern ancestry: Semiramis (Mixed Arab European), and two White or White-passing Jews, Romi (Moroccan) and Nava (Israeli). Then come the two participants who'd been born and/or are living outside of the United States, Aleks (Russian Armenian born in Azerbaijan and living on the East Coast of the US), and Fabia (Spanish-born, living in the United Kingdom). And lastly, I address the remaining seven White U.S.-born participants insofar as their racial identity had been something that they'd addressed during our interviews, which had predictably been less salient as Whiteness, as a sociocultural construct, still problematically operates as a presumed and unexamined background of neutral, universal, unchallengeable normalcy.

Black Mothers

The Black women (the Black women study participants had preferred that term over "African American" or had held the two as equally preferable) whom I interviewed had more to say about race and racism than any other subset of my interview participants. Throughout their incredible stories, they'd woven the threads of how both race and racism had strongly impacted their experiences of pleasure during birth, both from within and from without. For most, an anticipation of racist mistreatment permeated the birth space like a pervasive mental and emotional static, which was louder for some than for others. They'd expected to experience racist negative bias from their healthcare providers, casual or malicious disregard, disrespect, and outright violation of their bodily autonomy. These expectations were founded on their own lived experiences, the experiences of friends and loved ones, and the well-documented realities of obstetric racism and violence that undergird the maternal health crisis for Black women in the United States. And so, these participants were holding the awareness of these issues and responding to them throughout their pregnancies, bracing for how they might be treated during birth, and strategizing appropriately.

Those expectations informed their reproductive journeys in terms of their prenatal care, childbirth preparation, and their choice of birth setting. Those who'd delivered in a hospital had strategically mitigated the abuses that they'd feared by having rigorously prepared for their births, by having educated themselves, and by having intentionally armed themselves with a support team to create a perceived field of safety. Others had consciously chosen to avoid the hospital setting, particularly if they had experienced obstetric racism or obstetric violence during their past encounters with biomedical healthcare providers. There'd been a wide range of ways in which Black women responded to racism in their birth approaches, as described during our interviews. On one end was Chandra, for whom the static had relatively been quiet during her hospital births (until she'd been subjected to mistreatment, pressure to undergo unnecessary procedures, the denial of her support person, and nonconsensual analgesia). And now, I want to delve into Chandra's story about her first birth.

I have already highlighted Chandra's essentially pain-free hospital births, which took place during the late 1970s and early 1980s, because they contain so much thematically, especially in Chapter 3. Here I focus on her views on both race and racism, and on how these forces had interplayed in her otherwise lovely birth experiences. As a reminder, Chandra was 19 and pregnant with twins in 1978. She had a wonderful experience of pregnancy, enjoying the process fully, free of complications. She spoke about race in her first birth explicitly naming the racism, respectability politics, and the barriers to choice that had been and are still involved in giving birth as a young Black mother:

> I initially wanted to have my babies in the birthing center in New York. And then when they found out that I was having twins [pause], New York law would not allow my twins to be born in the birth center. So that was a big disappointment. That's why I had to go through that pattern of finding the right OBs, and then firing people who were not positive and affirming or caring, wouldn't look you in the eye. Or, you know, doctors who, you go to the obstetrician's office, and they see a young Black woman, and the first thing they do is they look down at your left hand to see if there was a ring on it. You know. I guess, fortunately, I was a married woman. And you could see their attitude shift immediately. And actually, I was treated respectfully, because I was a married woman. So, I'm sad for the women who walked in there and didn't have rings on … so that didn't feel good to me. But Dr. Cohen's office was a love fest. He's a sweetheart. He was real old school doc and one of those—he should have been a midwife.

To navigate the racist and classist respectability politics that she faced, she leveraged whatever strategies she could. Respectability politics (Higginbotham, 1994) is a term for the strategies that members of marginalized groups, especially Black people and Black women in particular, use to mitigate racist and classist oppression in the context of White supremacy; these strategies often involve conformity to the behaviors and appearances associated with, and therefore deemed respectable by, the dominant, namely White, group. To Chandra, the strategic circumvention of racism in the birth space had looked like preparation, planning, and teamwork. This circumvention had in part involved having drawn on her relationships with White men. She was married at the time to an educated White Jewish man. Also, her doctor, with whom she had a wonderful, supportive, and holistic relationship, was also a White Jewish man. She'd talked about this process as having been fundamental to her pleasurable birth experience, particularly as a survivor of childhood sexual and physical abuse:

> Being sexually abused and emotionally abused and battered, your self-esteem is in the toilet. And so, to be chosen to have two babies grow inside you was a really big deal for my little soul. I consider having my children the first big piece of recovery for me around how I was raised. And my commitment to be a different kind of mother, a better kind of

> mother, not a hurting kind of mother, was like really cemented in that pregnancy. *I felt good.* I gained really good weight. I bounced around. I was 19 too so that was helpful. But, you know, I didn't have doctors telling me a whole bunch of scary stuff. I fired doctors until I found a doctor that was more in line with my attitude. And I found a very nice kind of elder doctor, Dr. Cohen, who just kind of looked at my history and said, "You're a healthy young girl with twins in your family, you're gonna do fine." So that attitude was really helpful. His exact words were, "We're gonna have a good time." And every time I'd come in for my prenatals, he was just very affirming. When I would come in from my appointments and he'd be "Oh! Here's our beautiful twin mom! Hello, how are you? How are those babies?" You know, and he'd be all excited about them and touch my belly and listen to them. And let me listen to them. And, you know, he was so full of joy. And I borrowed that from him. It helped me so tremendously. I never heard anything negative from him. And if I heard negative something from somebody else, and I'd call him, he'd say like this "Who are you listening to? Don't talk to those people." [Laughter both]. So, I really, really—Dr. Cohen, may you rest in peace, you are a beautiful man, oh the perfect, perfect, perfect OB for me when I was having my babies.

Chandra's labor onset was subtle and pain-free, and her entire labor was only punctuated by occasional moments of pain, almost entirely due to certain people disrupting her dreamy head space with stress, triggering upset and fear. In the absence of stress or fear, her first birth in the hospital had been blissful and serene. Her first birth, with twins, started roughly 10 days past the estimated due date. As I've described in Chapter 3, and to recap here, Chandra had awakened in a dreamy, blissful state and had realized that her water had broken, and then, had called her mother to tell her that she might be in labor:

> I call my mother and I'm like, "I think my water broke." She screamed so loud that she scared me to death. "Oh my god! Where's your husband!? Are you alone?! What are you doing!?" So, I burst into tears. And she's like, "Oh, no, I don't mean to scare you. I'm sorry. I'm sorry. Sorry. It's okay. It's okay. You're gonna be okay."

So, this was the very first time that Chandra had felt uncomfortable in any way during her labor. Once she'd settled back down, she got her birth plan moving. She contacted a neighbor who had agreed to drive her to the hospital, she relaxed again into her feel-good birthing head space. In transit and when she got to the hospital, Chandra maintained this state. In terms of her birth preparation, she had anticipated some of the issues that she might face at the hospital and was not thrown off terribly by them. In her words:

> We had had our childbirth education at the birthing center we had initially planned to have the kids at, and they had warned us of the various shenanigans that hospitals might pull. One of the things they did—were trying to do in the early days, was that they would engage the husband in paperwork, and then separate the spouses, and then he'd be sitting for hours and could possibly even miss the birth because no one tells him to go to be in, and you end up birthing without your partner. So, they did that. They separated him into the office. And I went up in the elevator. I still wasn't afraid because I kinda knew that was gonna happen. And at that point, there wasn't like early registration thing, he had to go fill out forms to admit me to the hospital. So, I knew like the clock was ticking on how long I wanted him away from me. Um. I'm still feeling really good.

As she was moved up to the Labor and Delivery unit, her mother's fears again took hold. As Chandra looked out of the elevator doors at her mother's face, it was the face of "abject terror," "like she thought she'd never see me again":

> I had a moment of doubt as to what was happening with me in my body. And in the elevator ride up, I had to like to recalibrate myself, because I had read a million books. I had taken the classes with the wonderful midwives who wouldn't lie to me … I had breathed into that, the fact that I really believed that I would know if something was wrong with my babies, 'cuz they're inside of me and we've been having a good time for months. And I knew them really well. I knew where everybody was. And it was kind of weird that it didn't hurt. But what you're gonna do? It didn't hurt.

When she'd arrived in the Labor and Delivery department, she'd been so calm that the nurses had not noticed her presence there or had misread her as not having been in labor, for around 15 minutes. Chandra had to walk over to them to alert them to her presence, at which point they launched into frantic action. That was when Chandra started to experience being treated in ways she did not appreciate:

> My childbirth class warned me that they were going to try to shave my pubic hair. So, I had to tell them not to do it. And this one particular

> nurse took great umbrage with this and was trying to fight with me. And I was like, "Wow, you really don't understand that you shouldn't be messing with me right now. Because you're upsetting me. You ruined my buzz. Because really, I was like, high, and you're ruining my buzz. And I know we don't need to do what you're trying to do. My pubic hair is not toxic to my children. And you should go away now." And she didn't want to go away. (Sucks teeth). So, I was not very nice to her. I did use bad language. And then she went away. And so, she told all the other nurses that I was this horrible, cursing, crazy Black girl (laughter).

The "shenanigans" did not end with this individual nurse. Chandra realized that, as she was warned might happen, she was being kept from her husband, the only support person she was allowed to bring into the birth space with her. During our interview, she recounted:

> I was like, "Where's my husband, please?" "Oh, he's doing paperwork. Bah bah, bah." I'm like, "Okay, I've been warned about you people. The midwives warned me about you." And so, I said, "No, I really need to have my husband right now. I need you to go get him wherever he is. He needs to be with me as we're having our children." "Oh, I'm sure he'll be here shortly." And I said, "You don't understand me." And I was getting angry. And I sat up on the little gurney there in the prep room. And I crossed my legs and I said, "My babies are gonna have to force their way through my crossed legs if you don't bring my husband here right now." He was there in 10 minutes. He comes running out, "Oh, I'm sorry. What's going on?" And I'm like, "It's not you. They were just doing their shenanigans and I had to get angry." And when I got angry, that was the only time I felt any pain in my labor. Because when I said about "the baby's gonna have to force her way through my crossed legs," I didn't say it nice and calm like I did just like now. I yelled. I looked this woman in the eye and yelled at her and sat up and crossed my legs. And the stripe of pain went across my belly. Because all the muscles were tightened up. I'm so sure. And then I felt so sad. And I was crying because I had been feeling so good. And I was wondering if that affected my babies. And if they were okay, now, you know, because nothing was hurting. And why should it start hurting?

I'm highlighting this passage again because it is so powerful. Having to fight with these nurses had not only disrupted Chandra's pleasurable birth, but had caused her to feel intense pain, both physical and emotional. Having to fight to decline such a simple and useless routine procedure as pubic hair shaving, which is now rarely done, and then to have to fight so hard to have her husband there to support her, each is one level of how her needs had repeatedly been opposed. Facing such opposition in a moment and in a place that should be designed around meeting the birthing person's needs seems antithetical to the purpose of giving birth in a healthcare setting. And for Chandra, as a Black woman, she needed her partner present, not only for comfort. It was a matter of safety. Denying her that support is a facet of obstetric racism. Obstetric racism shows up in the casual enforcement of obstetric routines and standard procedures in ways that disrupt what might otherwise have been perfectly lovely. During our interview, Chandra shared:

> [At last] my husband was there. And he was very on point. It was a really good day for him. That was actually a beautiful high point in our marriage where he was totally there, once he was allowed to be there. And he was very loving, and talked nice to me, and put his arms around me, and rocked me, and the discomfort went away. And he was like, Papa Bear now like, "What's going on?" "What's the next step? What are we doing?" And I told him about how they wanted to shave my pubic hair. He was like, "That's not necessary." "Okay, we've already determined that." [Laughter] So he totally backed me up. And that's an important thing, too, racially. I'm in a room full of White people. My husband's a White person. And so, it is very important to feel allied in that way. You know, nobody was being overly racially anything but energetically that's in the room at all times. And so, here's a little Black person—well, a young Black person standing up for herself. My husband's a decade older than me, and a White guy, and all these White people. And he's got a degree. I didn't get my degree yet. [laughs] You know. All these things matter. So, people did put their noses in the right direction when he was there. And that was very helpful. Other than the fear from my mother, and other than the pain of having to argue with that nurse, I had no other discomfort having my kids. At that point, with my partner with me, I was able to relax. And I felt a need to push. And they wheeled me into the operating room, and they said, "Oh, you're complete!" So, this is all within a half hour of walking into the hospital, 40 minutes walking into the hospital. And then I think I pushed for another 15 minutes, and [Baby A] was born.

The delivery of [Baby B] had taken longer than it should have, partly because her biomedical care providers would not allow her to get up off of the delivery table to walk around. With conversation and informed consent, her doctor performed an internal version maneuver to reposition the second baby, who'd been in a posterior position, to rotate and better engage the cervix. Shortly thereafter, he was born, also vaginally. It was after this second birth that Chandra endured the most disturbing act of obstetric violence of her entire birth experience:

> The babies would put in the—in their little tubs and I wasn't able to touch them right away. I could see them. And I was like itching to have them. I was like "Please, I want my babies—can I have my babies?" And this stupid nurse comes up and she's like "You must be tired." And I'm like, "I'm not tired. I just really want my babies." And she's like, "Well, after you what you've been through, you must be tired." And like, "I'm not tired. I'm fine. Can I touch my babies? I haven't touched them yet." [Long pause] And then I'm looking into the buckets trying to see my babies and out of the corner of my eye I see her inject something into my IV bag, and everything goes black. She's knocked me out.

Being unwittingly anesthetized without consent is an act of extreme and completely unjustified obstetric violence. When she emerged from the effects of whatever medication had been non-consensually administered, she was furious:

> Baby B was born by 12:10pm. And his brother was born 26 minutes earlier. I woke up at midnight that night. So, I missed my children's whole first day on the planet outside of my body. [Long pause] So I wake up at midnight and I'm furious. I'm a furious fucking psycho 19-year-old Black Brooklyn girl; that's an ugly thing. I mean, you should be frightened to hear that. That should frighten anybody! I was so mad. And I just started raising hell like, "I want my babies!" At that time, people were just starting to breastfeed. So, the babies were in the nursery anyway, and they're brought to the mothers every three hours in little buckets. And I said, "I don't care." They're like "The babies are not ready to be brought out now." Like "I had those babies this morning. It's night. It's night the next day!—'cuz we're talking about after midnight. And I had these babies around lunchtime. I want my babies! You get them. You bring them to me right now!" [chuckles twice]. And I made such a stink that they went and got like the head of nursing to come talk to me try trying to convince me that I shouldn't ... uh ... have my own offspring! She was like, "Okay, okay, we'll get the babies for you. We'll bring them to you." "Hello?! Why was this even a conversation?" And why did that horrible—[pause] To this day I feel fury in my body about that nurse.

Most of her first day with her newborn children had unjustly been stolen from her. This theft is yet another profound act of obstetric violence. Once she'd finally gotten her babies back, everything had shifted for her. She relished in her babies, began their breastfeeding relationships, and felt overwhelmed with gratitude for her two beautiful children:

> So, they brought me my babies and the first thing I did was like I unwrapped them and held them and rocked them and kissed them and smelt them. And felt their little hands, and their little faces, and counted their fingers and toes 'cuz that's what you're supposed to do, make sure they have all their parts, which they did. They were so cute. And I was apologizing to them. Like "Mommy's so sorry that you were away from me. I love you. I didn't want to be away from you." And they were like "It's okay, Mommy." [chuckles] They didn't know any better. But I'm like that must have not been okay for your little newborn selves. Because my heart was broken. I can only imagine what their hearts felt like. And I just—we all got into bed together and I snuggled with them. So, we reestablished our connection and we were able to do that especially when I got out of the hospital. But, um, and I just spent that night and early morning just in in tears and gratitude. Because they were so perfect. These two beautiful golden babies—they were just perfect and I had made them and there was nothing wrong with them. You know?

Chandra's account of birth pleasure for a first-time mom of twins, as a young Black woman, provides a powerful foundation for the examination of race around birth, stripped in some ways of complications and medical interventions that can tend to obscure the baseline ways in which biomedical power is exercised over Black women's birthing bodies. When I asked Chandra what pleasure is, she replied: "freedom from fear—that I am … in an environment where I'm not afraid." And therein lies the rub. How to give birth free of fear as a Black woman in the United States? If Chandra is on one end of a range of experiences of fearful mental and emotional static, on the other end might be Malika, for whom the fear volume was at maximum levels. Malika had negative expectations about hospital birth based on what she'd already known and had heard, specifically about obstetric racism. These expectations had led her to choose an autonomous birth center to deliver her baby, but that had not worked out for her:

> I remember it like it was yesterday [chuckle] … I was prepared for birth, because I had a doula. And I had a bonus doula during the birth experience. We had a birth plan. And I say, unfortunately, because

> I really wanted to stick to the birth plan. But it was fortunate because things happen the way they're supposed to happen. I wanted to have my birth experience at a birth center. But because I had meconium—I think that is how you say it, I always mess it up—I wasn't able to have the experience at the birth center in San Francisco. And instead, I was rushed to SF General ... And I really, really did not want to have a baby in the hospital because I had heard so many bad stories, nothing was positive for African American women. And I was just so scared! Like, I'm scared right now—I'm about to cry. Because I've heard so many bad things that happen to the Black women, that they've neglected or not heard. And I really, in general, like, people in general are not heard at all. And—and I guess you can kind of tell what's happening in now in the, with the protests and stuff [speaking about the George Floyd protests]. But basically, they're just protesting because they're tired of not being heard or not being seen as a person. And I really did not want that to happen in my birth experience.

Malika's birth experience had been unusually long, spanning five days, and most of it had been both agonizing and exhausting for her. But she had not wanted to give up on the vision that she'd had for her birth:

> I really wanted to do everything natural, because I wanted to prove that I could. And it was a five-day labor because I was really stubborn. And I really wanted to make sure I had the birth experience that I really wanted. Yeah, so that's, and then on the on the fourth day, I was just my body was just tired, tired of laboring because it was like, it would start [and] it would stop the labor.

The fearful, negative thoughts in Malika's mind were major impediments to her having been able to relax into her birthing process in the hospital:

> ... the thoughts of "Are they going to hurt me? Am I going to be okay? Gonna hurt my baby? What are they going to do to my baby?" You know, those are the thoughts that were always going through my head. And I didn't really, I didn't necessarily voice it so that they can understand. But I did say a couple of times when they when they asked me, "How come I didn't want to take the drugs?" and all these different things. And I was like, because I didn't—I do remember saying "Because doctors are not great to African American women." I remember a couple times saying that.

There had been just moments of reprieve from her fears, one of which had been the special moment that Malika reported having been pleasurable during her entire five-day labor: a comforting experience with a doctor who'd also been a Reiki practitioner.

> I just I like remember hearing like the voice—it was the sound of the woman's voice. I felt like it was just me and her only in the room. She did ask me questions about my childhood. And I did cry. Because I guess it was so, so, so touching or so personable or so tender still, that I had, that that was the emotion that came out. And I just remember the voice, and just feeling like, you know, it was it was okay for me to go through what I was going through. "I'm safe. I'm okay." That's, that's pretty much what I was feeling.

When Malika had been less gripped by her fears, she'd been able to feel supported, and she had then finally been able to relax into her birthing process more, which made her experience less painful and more pleasurable. Voicing the many layers of their experiences had been a struggle for most study participants, who'd often found themselves grasping for words during our interviews. Malika had eventually found her own ways to put her conflicting birth experiences into words:

> I think the only time that I felt really good was during the Reiki exercise, and maybe giving birth because I, I wasn't worried too much about it. I knew that there was like a circle of midwives, doulas, and then doctor that was around me. I could feel their presence. I was kind of like still coming out of the epidural state. But, but I could feel that they were there, and they were there encouraging me ... I learned to try—to try to breathe like I'm in a wave. Yeah, it was kind of cool. [laughs] Yeah, that was a really cool, pleasurable experience. Like, I felt that—I felt that like I was in a wave. [laughs] ... It was just a wave that was just steady-flowing. So that I could be able to imagine that the baby's coming out in a wave. I don't know. I think I had to imagine the experience in order for the experience to happen.

In this way and in many others, fear is a major impediment to pleasure. No doubt racism and the associated fear of maltreatment, along with the array of potential maternal health outcomes inequitably heaped upon Black women, are valid parts of that fear pattern. Despite her best efforts, her careful preparation, and the support that she'd consciously rallied around herself, Malika's original birth plan had gone awry, and both her fear and pain overwhelmed her birth experience.

Similarly, Callie also prepared for and managed her birth with great intention, to avoid as best she could not only the challenges of childbirth but also the racism that she was expecting to encounter. As a reminder, Callie received an induction due to preeclampsia at 36 weeks. Her labor was fully induced from 0 cm with Pitocin and then a foley bulb was inserted after an epidural was placed, which was overdosed in error and caused many issues, including altered consciousness and headaches. Nonetheless, Callie reported having felt "peaceful" and "Zen," having consciously used her meditative and breathing skills throughout labor. She'd also used vision boards, music, and her community to build an ambiance around herself that made her feel safe and supported. As a Black woman of high socioeconomic status and high education, she brilliantly leveraged privileges associated with her and her teams' status and connections to protect her from the baseline racism that she acknowledged as endemic to the US healthcare system, particularly maternal health care. During our interview, she explained:

> I had these two doulas that were like rotating shifts. One who is an anthropologist, one who is a nurse. And then I think also relying on—relying on those identities [for leverage/power in the birth space]. And the anthropologist, the nursing staff at the hospital had Googled her. So, she was kind of a celebrity, which was helpful. They had, they had Googled me, and I was really surprised, but I should probably stop being surprised by like, students or mentees or folks in the healthcare professional profession, like knowing about me. So, my doula encouraged me. She was like "Use that, like, that's your leverage. Even if you don't want to, lean on that hierarchy or that power, use it to your benefit at this stage." My other doula who's a nurse knew many of the nurses in the hospital and was able to kind of relate to them as a peer but also as an outsider because she doesn't work at that hospital. So, *we used all of that.* [laughs] Yeah, we used all of that.

Callie also ensured that she had a very tight relationship with her obstetrician, who was Black and a sorority sister from the same college. Thus, she felt that her team had her back completely, which gave her the space to release fear, relax, let go, and drop into the experience of her contractions and her birth from a place of "Zen." As a Black woman, she'd, of course, been very aware of the perceived levels of risk that the biomedical system had assigned to her, having been categorized as "high risk" for her age (40+), her race, and her larger body size, that had hovered in the background as worry and fear. As someone who is very conscious of the risks associated with Black maternal health, specifically regarding her diagnosis with preeclampsia, she'd wondered:

> Being a Black woman giving birth over 40. Being in a city that has a lot of data, I guess, about the maternal mortality crisis and a lot of advocacy around it, I always—just wonder how I fit in that narrative ... even though I push back around the label of risk that sometimes—often is just lumped on Black Women, I am very conscious of like, "Oh, well, like how bad was it?" [for me]. Like, was it more dangerous and scarier than I thought? And maybe that's good that I didn't know at the time. But what does this mean?

And in the process of receiving this preeclampsia diagnosis, Callie had consciously engaged with the issues of racism and of dealing with risk factors:

> I always go back to racism because I'm a Black woman. Because I'm of a certain weight, because I'm a certain age, like, it's just assumed [that I had high blood pressure]. I don't have high blood pressure. Um, I've never had high blood pressure. And even after these two blips on this [prenatal blood pressure readings around 36 weeks], like, five minutes later, when they checked me, it was normal. And so yeah, I mean, I want the clinical staff to be vigilant, but I also don't want these assumptions made about like, "Oh, yeah, are you this [hypertensive] anyway?" Without even like, "Look, if you look quickly at my chart, you'll see this," or if you ask me, I can tell you without you just making an assumption.

So here, Callie draws attention to how racist presumptions of risk in certain health markers curtail the detection of real problems. And keeping full information from birthing people about negative risk complicates issues of both bodily autonomy and informed consent, particularly when fear is to be avoided for the sake of maternal wellbeing. Still, risk was not the predominating aspect of her racial identity that imbued her birth experience. She ensured that she was surrounded by Black people who saw her, cared for her deeply, and fully celebrated her. She had her team, her vision board, her two doulas, her husband, and her music. In her words:

> Our doula had asked my husband and I to make a collage together, a vision board of what is our, what was our vision of pregnancy and of labor. And so, we had framed that and had it up in the hospital room the whole time. It was in there, but it was facing me when I was

> pushing. And then my husband is a DJ, and we had a "Push" playlist. Now remember, I gave birth a month before I thought I was gonna be, so it wasn't mixed and scratched the way that we had thought, the planner in us, but we had a list of songs that we just shuffled. And during pushing, Destiny's Child "Survivor" came on [laughs]. And it was just perfect. Um, and you know, the nurses and the doctors were like, "You're doing great." And Survivor was on. I put up my Black Power Fist. And they were laughing. And then she was out, soon after that, and like, on my chest ... I remember just being really happy. Um, in the pictures I look like I'm crying. But I know, like, tears of joy. I felt really powerful. I felt really strong. And magical. Yeah, and like, "We did it!" We, me and her. And then we—like this village, this team that I have cultivated and conjured.

Personalized care, again, comes to the surface here, but in the context of race, that is seen in the full engagement and indeed celebration of Callie's Blackness during her birth experience. Her racial identity had been a part of what had given her birth its joy, its pleasure, its aliveness, even while there were difficulties and discomfort, even pain. She beautifully asserted:

> Birth can be pleasurable. Birthing people can define what pleasure means for them, and should define what pleasure means for them before, during, and after birth, and the complexities and complications of birth does not mean that that erases pleasure.

Here Callie teaches us that race is not risk, but that racism is, and that fear and even unforeseen complications do not have to steal the pleasure and joy from birth. Strategically planning for what will bring peace and joy, and bringing that into whatever birth space one enters, is a way to move toward pleasure in birth and away from fear.

Next, I delve into the birth experiences of the three Black study participants who'd avoided the hospital altogether. These women had surrounded themselves with affirming care, for many of whom their racial identity had been an aspect of this comfort. Sankofa, Callisto, and Melissa (Black and Latina) had all given birth at home. For Sankofa and Melissa, their home births had followed previous traumatic hospital births that involved nonconsensual procedures, biomedical mistreatment, and generalized disrespect that is socioculturally attributable to obstetric racism. For example, Sankofa's nurses had repeatedly put on the Grammy's on the television in her birthing room, despite her repeated clear requests not to. Her sense of the rapid progress of her labor had been patently and also wrongfully ignored. She'd been forced into painful birth positions by these nurses, and her pain and her clear verbal protests had completely been disregarded. She had been forced to accept a urinary catheter that she had not needed or wanted. The nurses and other care providers hollered at her "Push! PUSH!!" when she had not needed nor wanted this kind of aggressive coaching. They'd even brought her the wrong baby to breastfeed. The onslaught of stressful, unnecessary, sloppy, harmful "care" and frank mistreatment in this hospital had led Sankofa to choose a home birth going forward. The last three of her five births were beautiful experiences in her own home. Similarly, Melissa's second birth and Callisto's first birth had been home births. All three were married, heterosexual women with relatively uncomplicated pregnancies. All three of them felt that their home births had been a reclamation of their power, and none of them would choose to birth in any hospital after their positive home birth experiences, major complications notwithstanding. However, Sankofa and Melissa had less to say specifically about race and racism during their home births, perhaps because racism ceased to be salient within that context. In a commitment to improve birth experiences for other Black women, all three had eventually entered birthwork in various capacities, as doulas, childbirth educators, or midwives. Of these three, Callisto had the most to say about both race and racism.

Callisto's interview in particular drew sharp points regarding the racial elements of her pregnancy and birth. She'd grappled with internal family dynamics that had been rooted in their race around the absence of any kind of celebration for her pregnancy, and of Black women's reproductive lives in general. During our interview, she recounted:

> I was so bothered by my mother's dejected feeling about my pregnancy because I had been having so many conversations with other Black women about the fact that when you're like—It's very rare for a Black woman's pregnancy to be celebrated. Because no matter what your class identification is, how many degrees you have, no one's excited about you being pregnant. Like we're not supposed to get pregnant. We're not supposed to reproduce, apparently, you know, like, since we have been—since we—since we—you know, moved beyond chattel slavery into other forms of slavery. [laughs]. No one's excited about our reproductive lives, you know, and so, I think it's just, you know, kind of sad and kind of disappointing when your own family is like, lukewarm about you being pregnant, when this is supposed to be like one of the best times of your lives, and you're not only changing your status as a mother, but you're like bestowing a title on to them that they've never had, if they accept that title.

As her mother had not been a particularly supportive presence regarding her pregnancy, of course she had not shared her plans with her mother or felt compelled to seek her guidance or her feedback on those plans. This sense of protectiveness about privacy entwined, in some ways, with Callisto's great value for bodily autonomy—that her birth was her and her husband's business alone, and no one else need be involved.

Other racial themes emerged from Callisto's interviews as well. She'd had a feeling of invisibility as a larger-frame Black woman navigating predominantly White spaces, while she had not easily been identified as having been pregnant. Then, once her pregnancy had become apparent to others, she suddenly was showered with attention and was being touched by (often White) strangers. Similarly, during her postpartum period with her daughter having been perceived as "cute," she experienced being interacted with more than she felt comfortable, and she connected these dynamics to racism and the presumed availability of the Black body to White people. To Callisto, White people were, in general, problematically presumptuous, far too quick assume that they were welcome and wanted in her space when, in fact, they were not. She contrasted this dynamic with how she believes that she would not be equally welcomed to engage in the same overly friendly and hands-on behaviors with White people or with their White babies. During our lengthy interview, she explained:

> I just think that there's a lot of racial and class things at play. And also, just the fact that we live in a very "White space," and we're being touched and—you know, my daughter—people are commenting on her hair already, and just, you know, stuff like that. And I'm just like, "Ewww, like, don't. Don't do that. Don't do that. Because I know that if I start touching your child, it's going to be a problem." You know? And I just feel like I still have, you know, different feelings about engaging with other people's children than let's say, the average White person who's very touchy-feely, apparently. I just know that if I start being that way it won't be received well, and that's just the way the cookie crumbles.

Callisto had completely owned the process of educating and choosing her path herself and had fully accepted all of the consequences of those choices. To her mind, no one else will bear the consequences of her choices, so what do their opinions matter? Engaging fully in her own agency had in essence been a praxis in birth justice, something that she'd openly discussed her resonance with:

> My orientation to feminism and to birth is recognizing that I subscribe to the radical reproductive justice framework. It's the right to give birth,

> the right to not give birth, and the right to raise children in healthy environments free from harm and, you know, fatality. And so, it's not just enough to be able to say I had a normal physiological birth or, you know, healthy vaginal birth. It doesn't really stop there. Because, yeah, I can have a great birth experience. But if my child is, you know, 8, 9, 10, 11, 12 years old and becomes a threat, then what? You know, reproductive justice goes beyond just the birth event itself. And birth justice is, is great, because it really highlights the work of Women of Color, specifically Black Women who are working to change the narrative about birth in this country, and to address the disparities in maternal health and infant health.

Thus, Callisto rounds out the connections among race, racism, and birth pleasure. The ultimate experience of pleasure during birth is an experience of birth justice—bodily autonomy and safety, freedom from fear, wellbeing, and community. All of the Black women interviewed for this study articulated these important themes, and where these themes had not been present, pleasure had not been either. In this way, pleasure might be a signpost on the road to birth justice, especially for Black women.

Latina/e/x Mothers/Birthing Parents

Melissa, Araceli, and Cande identify as Latina/Latin/Latine/Latinx in a variety of ways. Melissa, whom I've also discussed above, is both Black and Latina, primarily identifies as Black mixed-race, and lives in New York. Araceli was born in Mexico City to a White mother and a Mexican father and was raised as entirely bilingual and binational. She acknowledges her White privilege, but culturally and ethnically identifies as Latina. Cande, a nonbinary person, was born in Southern California of Mexican Mestize descent and specifically identifies as "Latin." Cande had been clear that they can pass as White and recognized that passing as White has afforded them privileges in navigating their gender through pregnancy and birth. Cande had given birth to their first baby in an autonomous birth center just months before our interview. When I had asked them about race, they'd responded that they knew that it had made an impact on their birth journey, but it was a bit unclear as to how. As Cande explained:

> I mean, yeah, obviously, it [race] has [had an impact]. But I think also more in like, the ways in which I think about parenting … I'm, I guess, lucky that I can pass as White. Most people have no idea that I'm Latin. And so that has given me a lot of privilege in my identity as being non-binary, but also my identity as a parent … then it's like my

> own like coming to terms with—accepting that privilege and accepting assumptions of the politics of passing. A huge role. And sometimes I leaned into it for both my like gender identity as well as my racial identity. But I would say it definitely played a role, for sure.

Still having been so close to their birth, just a few months postpartum, Cande had not fully processed the ways in which race and racism had impacted their birthing experiences. But during our interview, they'd shared with me about how they have grappled with their own reclamation of their Mexican, Spanish, and Mestize identity, which had previously been something of a mystery to them as they were being pushed into the American "mainstream" and had lost touch with their cultural roots:

> I think maybe subconsciously I did make a conscious decision to like to go against the mainstream … I'm very much claiming my cultural heritage where like—mostly, I think it was unknown. Which is like this whole history within my family. My grandma had a different name that we didn't find out about till she was like 55. And there were certain cultural things that we did that I just assumed was due to location, not because of actual like, ethnicity. And it was very much, in my family, a push towards mainstream, whatever mainstream means. And so, like for me, it was like a reclaiming of the Mexican, Spanish identity. And the Mestiza identity within that. So, in that regard, yes. And I think mostly because of the big assumptions of community and culture, and in sort of more or less like US culture, I guess. I don't know if that makes sense.

During our interview, Araceli had also shared with me this same awareness of her White privilege, culturally passing as White, having a White mother, but having been raised as middle-class in Mexico. She'd had much to say about the tensions around her cultural identity, racial identity, and her approaches to her two births (both of which had taken place in a hospital but had been two very different experiences). During our interview, explained:

> I am Latina. But I also have the White lady power. That I feel like I can just ignore the medical system. Because I have the power. Right? And I have an advocate, my sister, who can also advocate for me and has the power. I don't think [her partner] who's Brown and Mexican has that power. Right? Or at least in the states he doesn't act like he has power. Maybe not in Mexico, because doctors are doctors, and you listen to them. Right? And so, if you're not White—if you're going to have a

> fabulous hospital birth, you really have to work really hard. If you're White, you have to work hard. If you're not White, because they're not—they're not organized for that—you have to work doubly hard, or triply hard, if you're not White.

Araceli was very clear that having been raised by a White mother, even in Mexico, had given her certain blind spots around race, and an imprint in terms of her birth culture, what she called a "hippie" birth culture. She explained:

> I do have blinders. Like my mom is a gringa. She had all her four children in a hospital in Mexico in a hippie way. Because she just did. She didn't do hypnobirthing, but she was like, unafraid. And like eating placenta and like nursing the babies at a time in the 70s were ... not—not what you did. Now, what you did in the States is definitely not what you did in middle-class Mexico. So, she had to fight, and it was like, completely 100% committed to, you know, the La Leche League and the hippie birth and all that. Even though they [the births] were in the hospital, she just like, had that. Plus, she tells stories that all her births—I don't think she was very sensitive to the contractions. Maybe she also had no fear. So, like they were all relatively quick. I have that as my like, my experience. And so, I have the blinders that come from being the daughter of a gringa. Right? A White gringa, not just—so whether anybody treated me differently because I was Latina, and they could see in my chart that I was Mexican, I don't think—I mean, like—I don't know.

This "hippie" birth culture had greatly differed from what Araceli would otherwise have identified with as a middle-class Mexican, for whom birth is hyper-medicalized. In some ways, her pursuit of a de-medicalized birth had been at odds with the Mexican culture, particularly the middle-class Mexican culture, with which she still identifies:

> I was raised speaking both [languages]. So that's why I say like, I have some of the blinders that don't necessarily happen with—but also, culturally, even though we didn't have much money, we had social capital. And so, we were raised middle-class. Right? And so middle-class Mexicans are all about medicalized interventions. I mean, Indigenous women have *partos* [births] and *parteras* [traditional midwives], and they like, know all the things, and they also have trauma. I mean, I'm not saying it's an idyllic situation because it's not. But they're more willing to have births at home, than—none of my middle-class friends. In fact, I think all my

> middle-class friends from elementary school had C-sections because they were at the convenience of the doctor. Like, like the 1950s in the US now, 10, 20 years ago. This is what it is in Mexico. So, I feel like I had my hippie birth because of my hippie Mom. I tried to have a [hippie] birth in the second one. But um, yeah, I feel like I'm not your average Latina. I'm like a transnational.

Here, Araceli draws a distinction between the Indigenous Mexican women who have, in her view, a culture that is familiar with and oriented toward de-medicalized birth and the "hippie" birth that she'd been raised to know about by her "gringa" mother. Together, these layers intersect for Araceli, in a complex dance of having fully been aware of her multiple White privileges, unsure about how she might have been "treated differently" as a Latina, and a critique of the middle-class Mexican culture that, again, she'd been raised in as having been (and continues to be) overly medicalized. Araceli's first birth was extremely traumatic for her. In some ways, she'd attributed the suffering of her first birth to having been overly reliant on biomedicine "to save her." When I asked her about how she identifies racially, she answered:

> Latina: that comes with like, a whole culture of people wanting medicalized attention, which I think is what influenced my first birth. Like, I am ultimately Mexican in that way, in middle-class and that way in Mexico. So like, "doctors can fix things." They cannot—they cannot fix your birth. But they think so. That's the brain, right? My mindset—I had both. I had my Mom sort of all her life telling me these things, but also, sort of Western aspirations, aspirations of Western medicine kind of culture.

During her second birth, Araceli had completely transformed her relationship with birth through a rigorous hypnobirthing practice, and ultimately had experienced a pain-free, powerful, liberating, and transformative birth experience in a hospital. Some of that, she knows, is because of her White privilege and her freedom to maneuver as she wished in biomedical spaces, which she attributes to that "White lady power" that she'd been able to access to protect her birthing head space. In these ways, cultural identity and pleasure connected for Araceli. An over-reliance on biomedicine, which is a common sociocultural phenomenon, had been a large barrier to her ability to experience a pleasurable birth, and her mother's "gringa" orientation had been perceived by Araceli as having been "an asset," in addition to the White privilege that she'd found had given her free license to pursue her own vision for her second birth.

Overall, all of the Latina/es whom I interviewed had firmly believed that their avoidance of racism had been key factors in their experiences birth pleasure. Those who were/are White-passing had access to White privilege, and they believed that this access played a part in how they were able to have a sense of safety and freedom in their births, and thus to experience pleasure therein. Melissa avoided biomedicalized spaces entirely by giving birth in her own home and thereby also avoided some of the fear that might have disrupted her pleasurable birth experience as a Black and Latina woman. Again, strategic management of the threat of racist mistreatment factored into their decisions, but in different ways than for the Black women whom I interviewed.

Asian/Pacific Islander Mothers

For the Asian/Pacific Islander participants whom I interviewed, race and racism were not particularly salient issues in terms of their experiences of pleasure during birth. To briefly reacquaint my readers, Raquel is US-born of Chinese descent who had delivered her firstborn baby in a hospital after having enjoyed a mostly pain-free labor, just a few months before our interview took place. Bree is a Vietnamese-born immigrant to the United States who had delivered her firstborn at home, pain-free, around two years prior to our interview. Dalisay is Filipina born and raised in the Philippines, who immigrated to the United States during her teens. She had delivered her most recent birth seven years prior to our interview, but it had been during her first birth, 19 years prior, when she'd had a profound spiritual experience, a vision of her father, which she'd connected to her Filipina cultural identity. She also discussed the impact of her Catholic upbringing, particularly as a facet of being Filipina, on her relationship to pleasure. Below I focus on Dalisay's interview because she went into greater detail about these cultural aspects and how they interrelated with her birth experiences.

In terms of her relationship to sexual pleasure, Dalisay cited her Catholic upbringing as a Filipina cultural phenomenon that she had been eager to break ranks with:

> I think that my social upbringing, in my family, my upbringing as a Catholic—and as soon as I turned 18, moving away from that, because I knew that was not for me as a woman. And for me—and I didn't know I was a feminist until later on so I wasn't associating my feeling of independence and wanting to move away from—from not only just some of the some of the social constructs of my culture, as a woman being Filipina, and all of those impositions of my rights as a woman,

> because of my culture and the—the gender roles that's being imposed as a Filipina. Those I totally took an about face, you know, as soon as I'm able to, which was when I turned 18. And same thing with the Catholic Church ... I discovered my, you know, my pleasure when I was 13 or 14, and felt a lot of shame around that, for discovering it. That— And so, I felt "Oh, this is gonna—" you know, the whole religion and cultural things, like, "I'm not supposed to feel pleasure," but I did. And I felt guilty every time I masturbated, you know, and all of that. So, thank goodness, in some ways that, you know, we lived in America, and I moved when I was 15, that I saw a whole different way of looking at things. I saw a different way of experiencing who I am. Independence that I feel that I can own. You know, after I became an adult.

Dalisay's willingness to embrace other ways of relating to her body had been connected to her bodily experience of pleasure during birth. But it had been during her spiritual birth experience of a vision where she'd seen her father in the face of her firstborn child that she'd connected to her lineage, to the gravitas of her grandmother, who'd been a healer, and to her aunties who'd also been healers, and who had tangibly related to the Spiritual World:

> I came from intuitive people. My grandmother was a healer. You know, in her village she actually was a midwife, but not a trained midwife ... She didn't know medicine, but somehow, she was the go-to person when someone was giving birth. And so, she birthed every single child in her village. I remember, during the summers in the country, she would always put together some kind of healing something—potion—she would like, heal—cure me. Over the years too, I would hear stories about my grandmother from my mom and from her siblings, about things that my grandmother did that no one can explain.

During our interview, Dalisay spoke at length about the spiritual practices she experienced as a young child in the Philippines. She was believed by her aunts to have been visited often by spirits who would make her sick. They would see these spirits and would then intervene:

> When I was a little child, I used to get sick a lot. And my aunts would tell me that it's because I'm being touched by ghosts, or spirits. And I used to wear these potions under my shirt—[they'd put them] by the door when I'd come to visit them because they knew that if I came, I would get sick, because there are spirits in the house. And I was a kid,

> and I don't know, somehow maybe it worked. Because I would not—you know, before, before doing these rituals I would always get sick. I wouldn't when I'd visit my aunts' or when I'd go to the countryside ... My aunt said actually one time she was meditating and then she woke up I was—I fell asleep on the couch—I was feeling sick again. And she said she looked up and there were spirits hovering over me. That's what she told me. So, then they started the process of putting talismans to ward off the spirits so that they don't touch me and hurt me. It's not that they're hurting me. It's that they want to connect with me. But I didn't know that what's happening with me—that I would just get sick ... I was growing up, and I think I believe it, because I would you know, growing up, I would feel like—like there are things—whispers and things like that around me. But it would always scare me—that—so I'd push it away.

This impulse is similar to her impulse to push away the vision that she'd had of her father just after her delivery of her firstborn. Dalisay was touched to have the opportunity to discuss her experiences with me and somehow integrate these experiences, to have them heard as valid and reframed as a memory of connection that she could treasure. In these ways, her culture, her identity, and her birth pleasure intersected. Her spiritual birth pleasure had its roots in very rich cultural soil. And the pleasure that she'd experienced during her first birth, now reclaimed, empowered her to reclaim more of those roots, those ways of knowing that perhaps defy the everyday reality that is given full validity within mainstream Western cultures. So here there is again, a reclamation of roots and a conflict with mainstream ideas.

White Mothers and Birthing Parents

The White study participants must be sliced through in a couple of ways to ensure that I've appropriately analyzed the participants' experiences in terms of their identification with "Whiteness," and beyond it. Three White mothers identified as White or mixed race and reported Middle Eastern North African (MENA) heritage, in part because they are White-passing, and second, because they wanted to be responsible for the White privilege they acknowledged as theirs. So, here I first attend to these White mothers/parent(s) in a subset of this section. Then, I address those participants who'd been born and/or are currently living outside of the United States, as their accounts differ thematically from those of the other US-born White mothers. Lastly, I turn to the White mothers who'd been born in and are currently living in the United States.

White-Identifying Mothers with MENA Heritages

This sub-section addresses White-identifying mothers with MENA heritages and identities. First, I want to explain to my readers why there is a MENA category in my analysis when my study recruitment numbers differ with respect to the quantitative counts done in the recruitment phase of my study. I'd been unsuccessful in recruiting anyone who had fully identified as MENA for my interviews. However, three participants who identified as White reported MENA ancestry. They were thoughtful about how they self-identified and were very aware of their perception as White-passing, and with it their White privilege. They were not comfortable adopting an identity label that would cast them as a "woma/xn of color." Hence, I am qualitatively grouping these people together because of a roughly shared category and because their stories had thematically differed from those of the other White interview participants. I want to be clear that when asked them about their racial identity, they identified as White, while they also specified their cultural and ancestral differences from a typical understanding of "Whiteness" in being Jewish (Moroccan or Israeli) or of mixed Arab European ancestry. Nava identified as a "White Israeli Ashkenazi Jew." Romi identified as a "White Moroccan Sephardi Jew." Semiramis identified as a "mixed-race womxn with White and Lebanese-Arab ancestry."

Overall, this group had more to say about their cultural and ethnic identities than about race and racism. They had not reported having experienced any obstetric violence or obstetric racism, which one participant had credited to her White privilege. During our interview, Semiramis had made little-to-no mention of either race or racism. She'd given birth in a hospital in Berkeley, California, and had a positive, pleasurable birth experience in some ways because she'd been fierce and unstoppable in that pursuit. Her approach to birth primarily indexes a rejection of the kind of "victim-mentality" that she'd observed in the White mothers who'd been around her growing up. These mothers had not wanted to talk about their births, having experienced birth as traumatizing, as she described:

> It was sort of hush-hush in our family. Like, "Let's just not talk about it," like, "This person had a bad experience, this person had a bad experience, or it was just like, horrible, or she was exhausted." And I was like, "I am not getting enough information about how to do this right. And I don't it want to be like that."

Semiramis's mother is White, European of Irish and Portuguese ancestry, and her father is Lebanese-Arab. At no point during our lengthy interview had she explicitly discussed how her mixed identity, White and/or MENA, had impacted her approach to birth or her experiences of birth, including how she'd been treated and/or mistreated by others during birth. But if she had a default culture about birth, it was the highly medicalized and White birth culture from which she consciously chosen to depart. Perhaps her mixed ethnicity had helped her to find some space between herself and the default and negative birth mentality she'd been exposed to as a child. I would assert that White privilege had played a role during her birth, as it had for all of my White participants. Semiramis in particular had felt free to reject medicalized routines in the hospital and to express herself with abandon as she moved through her birth process. As a reminder, she felt that she'd been labeled as "a wild one" and a special nurse had taken her on one-to-one, almost in a doula capacity. This latitude, this freedom of expression, and this responsive approach to care are not equally granted across all racial lines.

Of the three participants whom I grouped in this section, Romi had the most to say about race, racism, Whiteness, and her Jewish culture. For Romi, her cultural heritage as a Sephardic Jew of North African descent, specifically Moroccan, was integrated into her reproductive journey in ways that are somewhat at odds with her life choices. How her culture had shaped her birth experiences had become salient somewhat later when, during our interview, she'd had the opportunity to process the ways in which her birth experiences had connected to her cultural identity and values. Romi is a woman who has invested a significant amount of work in analyzing her racial and cultural identity through a Jewish feminist lens. She'd written a dissertation on the topic of the Jewish mother–daughter dyad. In this scholarly way, she had engaged with her identity before having experienced birth. Over the course of her reproductive journey, she has grappled with passing as White, with leveraging White privilege, with the "Whitewashing" of her identity, and with how her roots have been made invisible. During our interview, she'd explained:

> I did like a lot of research—minored in Women's Studies. And my dissertation was about Jewish female identity and the way it unfolds, like in the mother–daughter dyad. And I talked a lot about the Jewish feminist experience, and kind of what that looks like, given that Jews generally from Eastern Europe are White, we have White-skin privilege. And so, as a result, our experiences, often just a little bit Whitewashed, right? Because it's sort of like "Okay, well, you, you've experienced this relative success as compared to minorities," which is true, we shouldn't be seen on the same level, but there's a unique experience there. And what does that look like? What do

> Jewish women's experiences look like? And they are unique, right? ... In college I was really involved in my Jewish identity. And I was a part of Jewish organizations. And I was also part of the women's student groups, but there wasn't like a place for me to sort of access my Jewish female identity. There was no space, right? Well, if you're Jewish, then you're just White. And then, you're just like, you know—we'll just brush your experiences aside with the White women. Okay, there's a there's a space for that. But I have a pretty rich history and my family. Sephardic, right? They're not White, right? And they come from Morocco and there's so much richness there. And there's so much to explore, and that you don't really see when you look at me. And so, how do I negotiate that? And it's something that I get to choose how to portray. So okay, there's the privilege of that. But then, there's also the isolation and that, like, you don't really know who I am. And how do I convey that? It's just, there's so much there.

Here, Romi is grappling with the intersections of race, culture, and gender, and how those identities can erase or amplify certain pressures, expectations, and limitations with regard to gender norms around motherhood and childbirth. So, for Romi, her racial and cultural identities shaped the larger context in which she built her family, but less so her approach to birth or her expectations of the birth experience. During the aftermath of her first birth, as Romi had interpreted her new status as a mother within the matrix of meaning of her culture, specifically via her mother's example of rebellion against the gendered limitations of their culture. During our interview, she explained:

> I come from my mom's family in Israel. They're really orthodox. She comes from nine generations of rabbis. And my mom is actually the first—my mom became a rabbi. She's actually considered the first female Moroccan Rabbi in the world, which is pretty incredible. And she obviously had to break from tradition with her family because they're religious, and she's like a woman rabbi, and it's like crazy. Like, they don't necessarily accept that. But I grew up and I was exposed to a lot of my religious family. And there was something so beautiful about the way of life. And now in retrospect, I'm like, "I could never be like—live in that world." But just this—there was like a simplicity and this devotion to having children and that life. And, you know, it was easier. Like, I'd probably have five kids, you know? I wouldn't have everything else, you know? And I feel like there'd be a lot of limitations on me. And I'm not saying I want that. But there is something so lovely about just

> like having kids ... It's so important to me—to raise them [my children] with a knowledge of their roots and their heritage. And that's, that is like my next purpose. You know, like, I'm raising them to know where they came from.

During her two hospital births, Romi had experienced a great deal of biomedicalization and of biomedical interventions into her birthing processes, although with a lot of support and with significant privilege, which she named. But she had taken no specific approach to preparing for or giving birth that had put her culture or religion in the foreground. She recalled her birth preparation classes at Kaiser Permanente as having been problematic in terms of how both race and ethnicity were portrayed:

> I even remember I took one of the birth classes at Kaiser and they had a video of different birth experiences. And it was like the White woman who went in, and she had her natural, amazing birth. And then there was a woman, a Latina woman, and her family didn't speak English at all. And watching—it's—I can't believe they're showing this to our class. And it was like, she—the doctors were like, "Well, you need to have Pitocin. Now you need to have a C-section." This woman, like, didn't speak English at all. And it was like, "Oh, my God! You see, like, the way you're treating this person?" I was really shocked by that.

Romi had observed that, during the childbirth preparation classes in which she'd participated, "Whiteness" had always been associated with "natural birth" and with "positive birth experiences," and had been visually portrayed as such. She also observed that highly interventionist biomedical birth management had been presented as "necessary" for People of Color by default, and that People of Color should expect to be ordered around by their authoritative care providers, told what is so, do as their told, and defer any agency they might have to their biomedical team. During our interview, she'd shared these observations with much anger in her voice, and with a clear awareness of how these types of maltreatment are perpetrated against People of Color. Furthermore, the fact that language barriers were not presented as critical to quality care Romi found troubling. She reported that the childbirth preparation videos she was shown at Kaiser portrayed English-speaking practitioners communicating in English to patients who spoke no English, and with no translator on video, which is profoundly problematic and unjust. Romi's recognition of the racist implications of this had struck me. Although her Whiteness and her passing as White had their benefits in the hospital, the Whitewashing and the erasure of her true complexity also marked her birth experience. During our interview, she explained how her own racial and class-based privileges had protected her:

> I definitely see that [privilege] in my own experience. Like the fact that I had this doula that I paid for, you know, and was there advocating for me, and we were demanding that we be heard and ... and [the doula] paying attention to [me] only ... Of course, like the White women are going to experience different treatment in hospitals.

And, as she explained during our interview, her doula had played a critical role in both of Romi's hospital births, so much so that when Romi emerged from the fog of her postpartum period, she sent a deeply culturally relevant gift to her doula. During our interview, she had insisted on reading the message and the song that she sent to her doula. Here is an excerpt of the most culturally illuminating part:

> [Reading from her letter to the doula] "When I think of my own strength during the labor as well as your ability to empower, I recall the *eshet chil*, which is the portion of the book of Proverbs that we customarily sing on Friday evening before the Sabbath meal. The song is generally translated as *Woman of Valor* and has been widely adopted by almost every Jewish community as a way to give honor to the mother or matriarch of the family. It is a song of gratitude and recognition, an ode to feminine strength and qualities. And according to the Jewish mystical school of thought, it is sung in honor of *Shalina*, the feminine Divine Presence, as a gesture of my gratitude, framed in artistic rendering of the *eshet chil* that I hope you'll enjoy. Thank you so much for being our partner and guide, and [for] what became a truly amazing birth experience. I couldn't have done it without a woman of such valor." And then, I included a quote from the from the song, "*An accomplished woman who can find her value is far beyond pearls, give her the fruit of her hands and let her work her works, praise her in the gates.*" So I'm reading that because I think that sort of captures kind of what she provided for me, and kind of what I hope to have again. She was my guide. She was so present. She allowed me to access that deeper part of myself. It sort of allowed me to reconnect with my roots. It's something I'm very connected with my identity and my culture. But it sort of brought that to life again.

This excerpt captures some of the spiritual aspects of Romi's two births; the most salient kinds of pleasure that she reported in her interview were directly tied to this doula's support. This doula's support had been indispensable to Romi, and was accessible to her in part or in whole due to her White privilege. Yet doula care is often out of reach for those who need it most.

Sharing about her own birth experiences postpartum had occurred to Romi as having been yet another site where she'd been washed over and/or erased within White upper-class birth culture in the US. Romi had also found that discussing her own births and struggles with motherhood with others had its own degree of silencing. During our interview, she explained:

> I think, and too many women, people, we connect on negative experiences, right? There isn't enough celebration of one another. We're not lifting each other up as much as we should be, I think. I tend to have a hard time being friends with people who are like, super competitive and not authentic. Like, I like people who are just, you know, it's like, just be real. Like, when I meet other moms, and they're not willing to talk about the challenges of being a mom, I'm like, "Really? This is real."

Some of this erasure may be rooted in cultural differences and communication norms between Jewish and non-Jewish people. Romi had named two communication patterns that she had experienced as having been "inauthentic": 1) commiserating on the negative experiences of birth and 2) a tendency to bypass or stifle discussion of the challenging aspects of parenting. What I understand from this statement is that Romi longs for honesty about all aspects of birth and parenting, not just commiserating on the suffering endured during birth, and not just portraying a rosy picture of parenting, but rather wanting enough space for all of it—for the celebration of pleasure and joy, and for realness about what is hard or painful.

Nava's experience had in some ways been similar to those of Romi. Living in Israel, she'd delivered her firstborn in a birth center in Lower Galilee. Her identity had a somewhat strained sense of place, heritage, and ethnicity. When I'd asked her during our interview about how she identified racially and/or ethnically, she answered with tentative language:

> I would say—so—You know, Ashkenazi? Sephardi? All of that. Um, so I would say Jewish Ashkenazi, because that does have an ethnic relevance. Right? And although partially Sephardi, I know because, you know, my grandpa was like sixth generation Israeli. So, we do have Middle Eastern roots, strong Middle Eastern roots, but I don't consider myself Middle Eastern because I was born and raised in New York. And I have such a mix, you know, European, my dad, European, Russian, all of that.

For Nava, the identity that she wrought from such a mixed ancestry was anything but simple. During the screening process for this study, when I'd asked her how she identifies in terms of race, she'd answered "White," and then, had specified some of these same details, while rejecting a MENA identity label. And yet being in Israel, having a baby there, and with a belief in having roots there, the Middle East was certainly part of her constructed identity. She felt connected to Israeli identity and built her maternal identity in tandem, in communities that supported her parenting journey. During our interview, she'd shared:

> I now feel like a part of this new, broader community of women who have been pregnant, and who've had babies, and who have babies now. And I'm in like, a bunch of WhatsApp groups and Facebook groups, and it's like, nice to have that.

There are other layers of Nava's identity, her interpretation of gender in terms of her pregnancies, and her political environment. During our interview, Nava shared about how Israel's mandatory military enlistment affects her and fundamentally contextualizes the reproductive lives of Israelis:

> I know that for a lot of people in Israel when they have boys, they think a lot about the political situation—because of the army, the mandatory draft here. And it's mainly men in combat, right? So that's like a really relevant societal thing that you start thinking about when you have kids. I haven't really thought about it as much yet, because I have a girl and usually women aren't in as much danger as men are here. But that's a big prevalent societal thing where people have kids here, you know, they hope that by the time their kid turns 18 that there won't be an army—there won't be a need for this mandatory draft.

In this way, Nana highlighted how Israeli identity and the militaristic Israeli culture intersect with birth culture, even several years prior to 2023 and Israel's ongoing campaign of genocidal violence against the Palestinian people in Gaza. Nava had also acknowledged that, within the context of Israel's healthcare system, out-of-hospital births are marginalized and therefore are inaccessible to many people. In this way, she counts herself as being privileged for having the opportunity to give birth in an autonomous birth center and is committed to advocating for others to have the same opportunity:

> Israel is such a mess as far as out-of-hospital births. There's no—insurance doesn't cover out-of-hospital births. So, it makes midwifery

> really expensive. Having home births is considered only for rich people these days because your health insurance won't cover a midwife. And, you know, we couldn't afford, like, in our current state, we couldn't afford having many more home births in the coming years because it's expensive. I don't know what it's like in the States, but it's really expensive, whereas hospital births are free, because it's subsidized. And I'm glad that it's free there but it's a shame that insurance doesn't cover midwives. I've become passionate about that. But I feel almost limited right now, because I'm just focusing on this [baby]. I think in the future when I, you know, have more time and sleep and all of that, then I'll hopefully get involved and hopefully, I'll keep the passion there.

In this way, Israeli militarism and healthcare access were both salient for Nava as she integrated her birth experience and her identity during our interview. In acknowledging privilege and constraint, freedoms and their denial, I find that there are parallels in how bodily autonomy is policed and managed by the State reflected both in the healthcare system and military conscription in Nava's interview. Bodily autonomy, regardless of venue, is shaped by structures of power.

Overall, the kinds of themes shared by these three participants are distinct in many ways from the other White participants that follow in this section. Their experiences of passing as White, identifying as White, and being "Whitewashed," combine with White privilege. Simultaneous sociocultural marginalization and erasure combine with Whiteness to produce a unique set of experiences for these participants. Although they were not subjected to any obstetric violence, particularly not on the basis of their racial identity, they still came up against the limits of bodily autonomy in the birth setting, specifically in the hospital where routinized care is normative (for multiple examples and analyses of such routinized care, see Davis-Floyd, 2022, pp. 90–186). These participants' conflicted relationships at the intersections of cultural identity, gender, and Whiteness stand out as compared to the other White participants who had not experienced such frictions, as also had the White-identified, born and/or living abroad participants whom I discuss next.

Two mothers, born outside the United States, have particular relationships with Whiteness and birth culture that warrant a specific analysis. Fabia is Spanish, born in Spain, and was living in the United Kingdom at the time of our interview. Aleks is Russian-Armenian, born in Azerbaijan, living in the United States. Both identify racially as White, and both are highly critical of hyper-medicalized birth, although in very different ways. Fabia's critique centers on sexism, and Aleks's critique is more intersectional, spanning gender, race, class, and sexuality. In terms of race and racism, these participants were quite different in their relationship to race as compared to the remaining White participants I interviewed. Fabia's interview revealed more about the cultural frictions between her current environment in the United Kingdom, which she found to be much more conservative and restrained than her Spanish cultural roots. Aleks, on the other hand, had a tremendous amount to say about race and racism, and spoke to these in very nuanced terms, as a sociology scholar whose wife is Black. Their relationship involves rigorous and vigilant awareness of White supremacy and antiracist practice. Aleks's most recent pregnancy and entire birth journey had, in some ways, been an antiracist expression. Due to the life-threatening health risks that Aleks's wife had experienced during their previous pregnancy (and would likely have faced carrying any future pregnancy, including the dangers of obstetric racism and violence), Aleks had insisted on carrying the baby. To protect their wife, Aleks became her surrogate. Aleks had intentionally leveraged their privileges as a White-bodied person who tolerates pregnancy well, free of the same kinds of impacts of racism: environmental, biomedical, obstetric, and beyond. During our interview, Aleks explained:

> I think about race a lot, in general, as a scholar of intersectionality, and as someone who's very attuned to health care being a very racist place and worrying about my wife's pregnancy being so different from mine. And the many ancestral traumas that she carried and experienced that led to her losing the child, and then led to me considering carrying again, because I wasn't—I was done at three. I don't know if you know this, but I was done after the 11 pounder. And I, you know, I'm very Russian in my thinking that I was like, "Oh, you know, you have babies in your 20s. In your 30s—that's for Americans." So, that's how I was. And then my wife tried and lost the baby and it—we grieved for a year or so. And then it dawned on me in the middle of a Pilates session, and an exercise session that I was doing at home, I looked at the mirror, which is how all my epiphanies come to me. And I said to myself, "I'm training to be pregnant." It was weird. I was like, "I'm exercising some [to] get my body strong for pregnancy." ... And it was like this whole shift. I was like, "I'm gonna carry your baby ... I don't know why we didn't think of that. I'm excellent at pregnancy. Just generally speaking, it's like, much easier for my body than for yours," you know ... It is an issue of race and inequality. Because, like so many Black women, she had a history of fibroids. Like so many Black girls, she had a history of poverty as well as having hair relaxing products, which also connects to fibroids, and actually causes issues with fertility, and it's part of like the way environmental racism contributes to maternal issues for Black

> women. So, we like pieced together her existence in the middle of these patterns and why she faced at each of the of the points what she faced, including her experience with preeclampsia and having high blood pressure and the way that her body responded … And the decision that we made to end the pregnancy was because I was like really aware of these inequalities.

Aleks had conceived through in vitro fertilization, had carried their wife's fertilized egg to term, and had given birth at home with the care team whom Aleks had believed would best honor their wife's identity, a queer Black woman midwife and birth team.

> I was just like, "Let me carry the baby." So, I think about race and inequality a lot when it comes to this. And also, when it comes to who gets to avoid the hospital and why and who gets to find midwives and doulas that look like them. Um, so not just—not just Trans and Queer people, but can Black women find midwives? And we did. We did find a Black queer woman midwife, but only because I went on the internet and was just like, "I need a Black queer midwife. Does anybody know one?" and was very explicit that way, and that's how, you know, you have to be, to advocate for people. And so, I imagined that my body was sort of a surrogate for her. So, if she were to give birth to this baby, this is the team that she would want. And so that's the team we assembled. It didn't matter that I was the vessel or whatever, I was just like "This is who would be your midwife, so ... this is who you would be your doula. So, we're going to do that. Because that's, you know, it's your—it's your baby." A miracle, a miracle baby. So, but in any case, those two frozen embryos on ice are—I'm still going to carry them. Like she's [my wife is] not going to be put through that again. There were doctors saying like, "She should try as her body's more used to pregnancy, and it won't respond that way" and whatever. And I was like, "No, we're not taking a risk like that again."

In these ways, Aleks and their wife navigated race and racism in their birth journey. It was openly discussed: obstetric racism was tackled head-on with strategic their team-building and by maximizing bodily autonomy. For them, this looked like avoiding biomedicalized spaces by delivering at home. Here, the major findings in terms of race had been their examples of proactive antiracist queer birthing, leveraging their White privilege for Black wellbeing within the context of a queer biracial relationship. It was not clear how Aleks's own identity in terms of race or ethnicity contributed to their birth approach, beyond the selection of certain birth comfort measures such as listening to ballet music. In their words:

> I took off everything, and I went into the bathtub, and I told her to give me the pregnancy ball, you know, the yoga ball, and to set up like candles and to be there with me and to put on ballet music—because I'm Russian so classical ballet music to relax me. And think it wasn't so much that I was connected to my wife, but like her presence, there is always like a very safe place for me. And so, it was more of that I was connected to my body in a very pleasurable way. Because I was just like, really in control. And I liked the music and the candles, and she fed me clementines, and it was like the way we always are.

The sweetness of this experience, the generosity and safety, and the intimacy are what stand out most. Their entire pregnancy and birth process had, quite literally, been a love letter for a queer Black woman, a gift, and an act of rebellion against White supremacy.

Seven study participants had reported no cultural or racial identity beyond Whiteness and had been born in and are living in the United States. As I've previously noted, and to recap here, overall, race and racism had not been salient for these study participants. Their White identity, in their minds, had little to do with the ways in which they had experienced their births, the pleasure therein, or the context within which their birth experiences had taken form. The main way that race was discussed by the White participants was in their identification of their own White privilege, while speaking to how they 'd benefitted or at least had been less subjected to the kinds of trauma and abuse that far too many People of Color experience during their births. Although there is little to quote in these interviews regarding race and racism from these White participants, I present an analysis of both Whiteness and racism as they pertain to these interviews.

There are generally two factions of Whiteness in terms of birth culture among these study participants. First, there are those who are critical of hyper-medicalization, who fit into a sort of counterculture of birth, advocating for "physiologic" or "natural birth." In terms of optics, this longstanding and still current movement trends toward upper-class White women, although, in some ways, the data that I've presented herein and also in other chapters challenge this stereotype. Some of these women had rigorously pursued childbirth preparation such as the Bradley method, Lamaze, Spinning Babies, or hypnobirthing—programs that have associated costs not all can afford, and are taught mostly by

White people. White people more often have the financial means to seek out doulas and midwives, most of whom are White; their services are not always covered by insurance, particularly not by public insurance (at least until recently in some places in the US). White people generally have more cultural latitude to participate fully in this kind of countercultural movement, even in rather conservative communities. White birthworkers therefore can be presumed to have more clientele to financially sustain themselves through their birthwork. While doing the very important work of resisting and transforming hegemonic technocratic birth culture through these countercultural practices, White privileges remain and reproduce themselves within birthworking spaces.

On the other hand, there are the White participants who adhere to medicalized birth culture, which, again, is the hegemonic and normative approach to birth. Hospital birth was historically crafted by and for Whiteness, and it is culturally safe for White people, a background against which Whiteness is invisible. Biomedical White supremacy is invisibly exalting of (certain normatively legitimized kinds of) White women and White births. Dorothy Roberts (2017) had been the first scholar who helped her thousands of readers to understand how eugenic policies had first been inflicted on poor White people. Expecting good and fair treatment in hospitals is an invisible (upper- or middle-class, educated, heterosexual, 20–30 something, thin, married…) White privilege. Even those who would prefer to avoid the hospital because they oppose biomedicalization and/or the kinds of oppressive dynamics that often pervade such spaces, may not have the luxury to opt out. These invisible privileges stack up: having care providers who look like them; who speak their language; who explain things in terms that they understand. White people do not worry if their care provider is going to be vigilant about and responsible for their own racist ideas and negative biases toward White people. White people have the luxury of generally trusting their care providers or not having palpable fear of them that Black and Brown people do not, although many thousands of White birthing people living in the US and also in many other countries are frequently mistreated by their biomedical care providers and are often subjected to multiple types of obstetric violence (Davis-Floyd, 2022; Liese et al., 2021). While I fear that these points are painfully obvious, they might not be to White people who may read this book, as these racial dynamics went unnamed within my interviews with most White participants. Yet the Black, Latina/e/x, and Asian participants had clearly articulated their experiences of race, racism, and the notable absence of White privilege, during their births, with varied and visceral depth.

References

Crear-Perry, J., Correa-de-Araujo, R., Lewis Johnson, T., McLemore, M. R., Neilson, E., & Wallace, M. (2021). Social and structural determinants of health inequities in maternal health. *Journal of Women's Health*, *30*(2), 230–235. https://doi.org/10.1089/jwh.2020.8882

Crenshaw, K. (1989). Demarginalizing the intersection of race and sex: A Black feminist critique of antidiscrimination doctrine, feminist theory and antiracist politics. *University of Chicago Legal Forum*, *1989*(1), 139–167. http://chicago unbound.uchicago.edu/uclf/vol1989/iss1/8

Davis-Floyd, R. (2022). *Birth as an American rite of passage* (3rd ed.). Routledge.

Easterbrook, M. J., Kuppens, T., & Manstead, A. S. (2020). Socioeconomic status and the structure of the self-concept. *British Journal of Social Psychology*, *59*(1), 66–86. https://doi.org/10.1111/bjso.12334

Higginbotham, E. B. (1994). *Righteous discontent: The women's movement in the Black Baptist church, 1880–1920*. Harvard University Press.

Liese, K., Davis-Floyd, R., Stewart, K., & Cheyney M. (2021). Obstetric iatrogenesis in the United States: The spectrum of unintentional harm, disrespect, violence, and abuse. *Anthropology & Medicine*, *28*(2), 1–17. https://doi.org/10.1080/13648470.2021.1938510

Nam, C. B., & Terrie, E. W. (2021). Measurement of socioeconomic status from United States census data. In M. G. Powers (Ed.), *Measures of socioeconomic status* (pp. 29–42). Routledge. https://doi.org/10.4324/9780429049170

Roberts, D. (2017). *Killing the Black body: Race, reproduction, and the meaning of liberty* (2nd ed.). Vintage.

Rolfe, S., Garnham, L., Godwin, J., Anderson, I., Seaman, P., & Donaldson, C. (2020). Housing as a social determinant of health and wellbeing: Developing an empirically-informed realist theoretical framework. *BMC Public Health*, *20*(1), 1–19. https://doi.org/10.1186/s12889-020-09224-0

Simone, N. (1965). Feeling good [Song]. On *I put a spell on you*. Phillip Records.

7

THE PLEASURE-FORWARD MODEL OF BIRTH

Oxytocin and the other happy loving hormones are not optional for us to be healthy.

Chandra

This study has revealed that pleasure and pain are both multidimensional and integral aspects of birth experiences, can co-arise, and are not mutually exclusive. It has also shown that birthing people who experience birth pleasure related to it in many ways, but to put it simply, had experienced birth pleasure either passively and unexpectedly or had actively pursued the experience of pleasure. Further, it has explored the ways in which relational, contextual, structural, and sociocultural realities had come to bear on the participants' experiences of pleasure during birth. These active pursuits had varied by person, based on their own social locations, their mindsets, and their orientations toward birth pleasure, their choices of birth support people and care providers, and how those around them had either enhanced or detracted from their pleasurable birth experiences. Although the causal relationships between the relevant factors that I have identified in this study have not been quantitatively tested, my qualitative data suggest that most factors flow bidirectionally and are nonlinear and reflexive within their complex relationships. I have coalesced these findings into a preliminary framework to guide practical applications and to frame further explorations: the Pleasure-Forward Model of Birth (Figure 7.1).

DOI: 10.4324/9781003499428-8

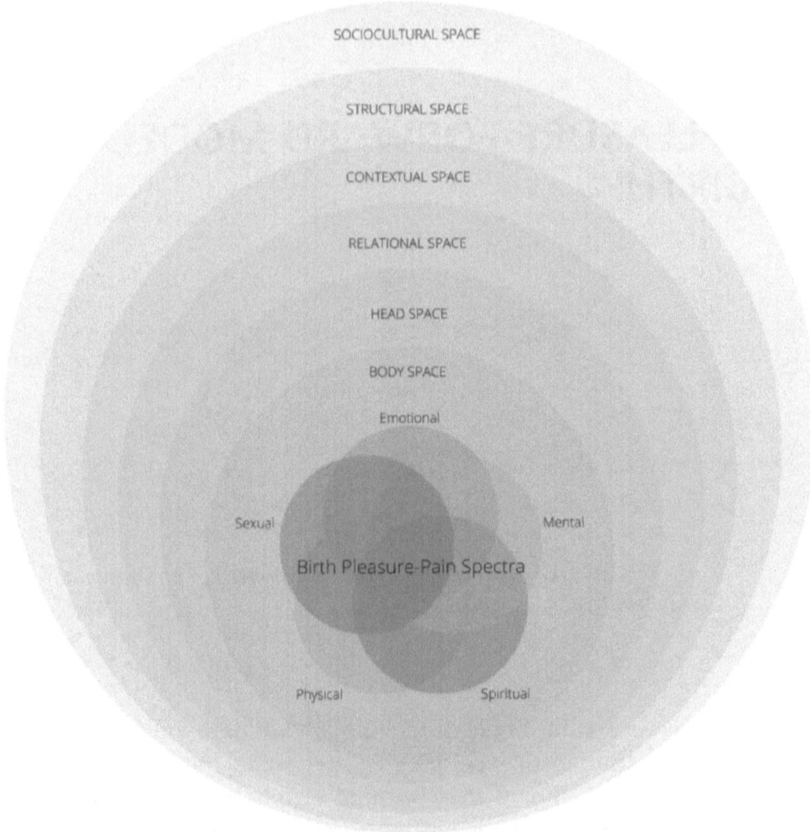

FIGURE 7.1 The Pleasure-Forward Birth Model.

The Conceptual Grounding of This Model

I've built this model from these mixed-method data, and standing on the shoulders of the many people who have devoted their energies toward improving birth, human wellbeing, and social justice from a number of disciplines. First, I honor as foundational the powerful frameworks of reproductive justice (Ross & Solinger, 2017) and birth justice (Oparah & Bonaparte, 2015), the ever-relevant critical pedagogical model of praxis (Freire, 1970), as well as pleasure activism (Brown, 2019) for contextualizing and dismantling the hierarchical and structural oppressions permeating and enveloping the birth space. I also borrow from public health mainstays such as the bioecological systems theory (Bronfenbrenner, 1974, 1977; Bronfenbrenner & Ceci, 1994), the biopsychosocial model (Bolton & Gillett, 2019; Engel, 1978), the health development model (Bauer & Jenny, 2007), and the salutogenic model (Antonovsky, 1996). I have done my best to create a model that is useful for the biomedical and midwifery models of birth care (Sandall et al., 2013), and have found Robbie Davis-Floyd's (2022) three birth paradigms (technocratic, humanistic, and holistic) useful for thinking about the ways in which theory, structure, and social forces interact in and on the birthing body. The *Listening to Mothers* studies lead by Saraswathi Vedam and her colleagues have provided tremendous insights into the mistreatment of birthing people, and into what is at stake in the fight against obstetric violence and racism (2019). I have also employed Roach's (2020) excellent ROOTT (Restoring Our Own Through Transformation) theoretical framework for Black maternal health inequities as an inspiring example of the critical analyses of the social and structural determinants of health, especially obstetric racism (Davis, 2019). Aligned with Crossing's (2021) work, I've also considered polyvagal theory (Porges, 2009, 2018, 2022) in my efforts to understand how relationality within its context imbues physiology, becoming embodied through neuroception (the unconscious detection of threat or safety) and coregulation (the mutual adjustment of actions and emotions among people) in ways that can either support or derail positive birth experiences and birth's physiological processes (more details to follow, and see Figure 7.3 for a visual guide).

Pleasure-Forward Model Constructs

Many layers of reality coalesce in and around the birth experience. In this model (Figure 7.1), I've used transparent layers of concentric circles to convey that these layers are not separate but rather permeate all aspects of the birth experience and are felt at each level. All layers are present and impact the birthing experience in ways that either enhance or diminish it. This Pleasure-Forward Model first envisions a particular birthing person's experience at the center of many interrelated and dynamic spheres of influence, much like Bronfenbrenner's (1974) biosocial systems theory and Jordan's biosocial theory of birth (1993), as mutually influential systems that are also structured upon both power and privileges. At the center are the birthing person's experiences and thus what I've called The Birth Pleasure-Pain Spectra, which was covered previously in Chapter 2.

The Birth Pleasure-Pain Spectra

This study's clearest finding has been that pleasure can certainly be a real experiential aspect of birth and can occur alongside or in the absence of pain. Pleasure is experienced in various modes and intensities, as is pain, and they are not necessarily mutually exclusive. I have depicted this finding as "The Birth Pleasure-Pain Spectra," modeling rich, overlapping, sometimes compounding experiences across the typology of pleasure that I have uncovered in this study: emotional, mental, spiritual, physical, and sexual (see Figure 7.2). I've used the plural "spectra" because, based on these data, I do not locate birth pleasure and pain on either side of a single spectrum. Rather, I see birth pain and pleasure as two overlapping, multifaceted spectra. Birth pleasure can be experienced in many ways, from not at all to a maximum intensity. Birth pain is also experienced on a spectrum, from not at all to a maximum level, and may well deserve its own typology, though I have not addressed that topic in this study. I have struggled with how to convey the fluidity, the circularity, the spiraling, the multi-tidal aspects of birth in these images. All seem to fall short of capturing the breadth, the aliveness, and the wonder of the birth process. Please forgive the flattened imagery, and if you can, recreate it in your mind in three dimensions or more, swirling, throbbing, and shapeshifting through time and space. All of it is in motion, all of it is permeable. All of it defies simplification. And yet here I am simplifying it.

Body Space

I have depicted the Birth Pleasure-Pain Spectra as central in what I call *body space*. I use *body space* to denote the birthing person's experiential and embodied self. It includes sensations, emotions, notions of "energy," and other interpretations and ideations about the birth process as experienced within the birthing body. It also includes the labor process itself, the various physiological functions, fluxes, and flows of birth. Body space is also the level of labor positions, vocalizations, and the physiological impacts of comfort measures like touch or water birth, as well as therapeutics, procedures, and medications. Again, see Figure 7.2 for a visual depiction of this construction of the birthing person, and their body space and head space (to be covered in its own section below) in relation to their experiences of pleasure and/or pain.

The interplay of mind and body is complex and requires some specific articulations. To better understand this interplay, I turned to biological literature. One potentially relevant framework that stands out is *polyvagal theory*, first in its concept of *neuroception* as an unconscious perception of threat and safety, and second, the role of nervous system *coregulation* for physiological response and emotional attunement with another within a shared context (see Porges' many works on this concept, starting with 2019). Porges argued that the physiological responses to danger at varied

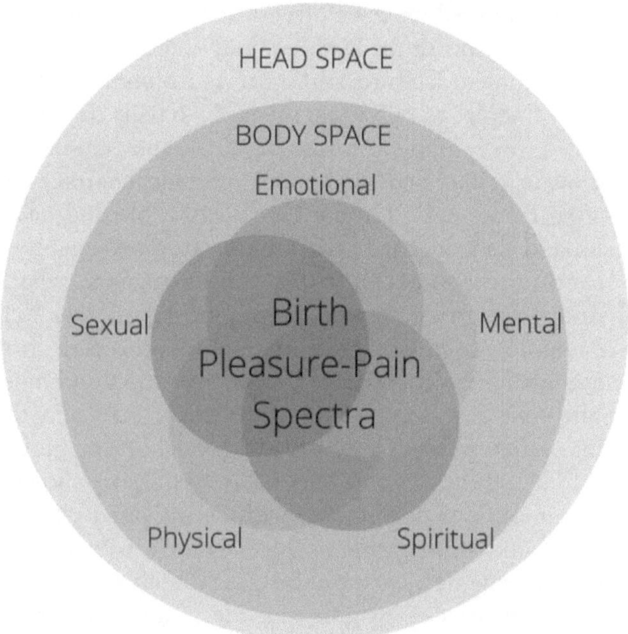

FIGURE 7.2 A Construction of the Individual Birthing Person: Body Space, Head Space, and the Birth Pleasure-Pain Spectra (as per the Pleasure-Forward Birth Model).

levels and within a social context are moderated by the different aspects of the vagus nerve, which is a nerve that is known for its meandering involvement in many bodily systems including the female reproductive system. However, Porges had not rigorously applied polyvagal theory to female reproductive physiology, birth included, at least not in a way that would account for pleasurable experiences of these physiological processes. For the sake of scope, I will reserve an expansive treatment of polyvagal theory and other related neuropsychological works for other, more collaborative, publications. For now, I offer that my study's findings and their resulting Model expand the range of birth experiences to be considered by Porges and others, and thus might affect the application theories such as polyvagal theory or other relevant tools from trauma-informed therapeutic modalities such as trauma-informed cognitive behavioral therapy (Yadav, McNamara, & Gunturu, 2024) or the use of techniques that modulate physiological arousal such as breathwork like physiologic sighing or non-sleep deep rest protocols (Balban et al., 2023) to birth physiology.

Polyvagal theory has offered me a way to holistically examine both the tangible and intangible aspects of the birthing body-mind, as situated as it is within relationality, context, culture, and time. As a humble start, I have applied aspects of my findings to polyvagal theory by having drawn on the works of many others (for example, Choi et al., 2014, and Schlote, 2021), which I present below in a simplified "dial-based" graphic that tracks threat activation levels (see Figure 2.1). I argue that pleasurable and pain-free birth indeed occur, and they appear to track best with polyvagal theory's construct *ventral vagal homeostasis*, or in less clinical language, what I am calling "Thrive Mode" (the green range in this graphic, Figure 2.1). "Thrive Mode" is where non-defensive biological and social processes—resting, digesting, healing, connecting, and other relaxed states—occur unimpeded. In this graphic, the yellow and red columns represent activated threat-responsive nervous system physiology: "Survive Mode" in the moderate, and "Shutdown Mode" in the extreme. My study has clearly shown that not all births occur in Survive or Shutdown Mode activated physiology, although the current and still-hegemonic birth culture overwhelmingly predisposes both of these modes. I want to be clear that this "dial" should not be construed as normative. I imagine that the ranges and thresholds between these two modes of threat response would be different for every birthing person, of course, depending upon their unique personality, health factors, birth history, beliefs, preparation, trauma history, sociocultural positionalities, and those of those around them. Supporting Thrive Mode physiology during birth could be more rigorously investigated as an avenue for improving birth wellbeing and maternal health outcomes. Based on my work herein, birth pleasure might be considered an indicator of Thrive Mode birth physiology in real time, much in the same way that an elevated heart rate is a physiological indicator of sympathetic activation within Survive Mode. But all of the above is as much a structural and cultural question as a biological one, as context is decisive in perceptions (and perhaps neuroceptions) of threat and safety, particularly for people who are presently facing the structural threats that racism, sexism, classism, and gender and sexual oppression all pose. These oppressive forces and obstetric violence likely further predispose certain birthing people toward activated threatened states that compromise their birth wellbeing, just as Chandra's, Sankofa's, Malika's, Araceli's, and Debbie's hospital births had so clearly revealed. (See Chapter 6.)

Head Space

In the Pleasure-Forward Birth Model, surrounding the body space is what I call: *head space*, the state of consciousness in which the body

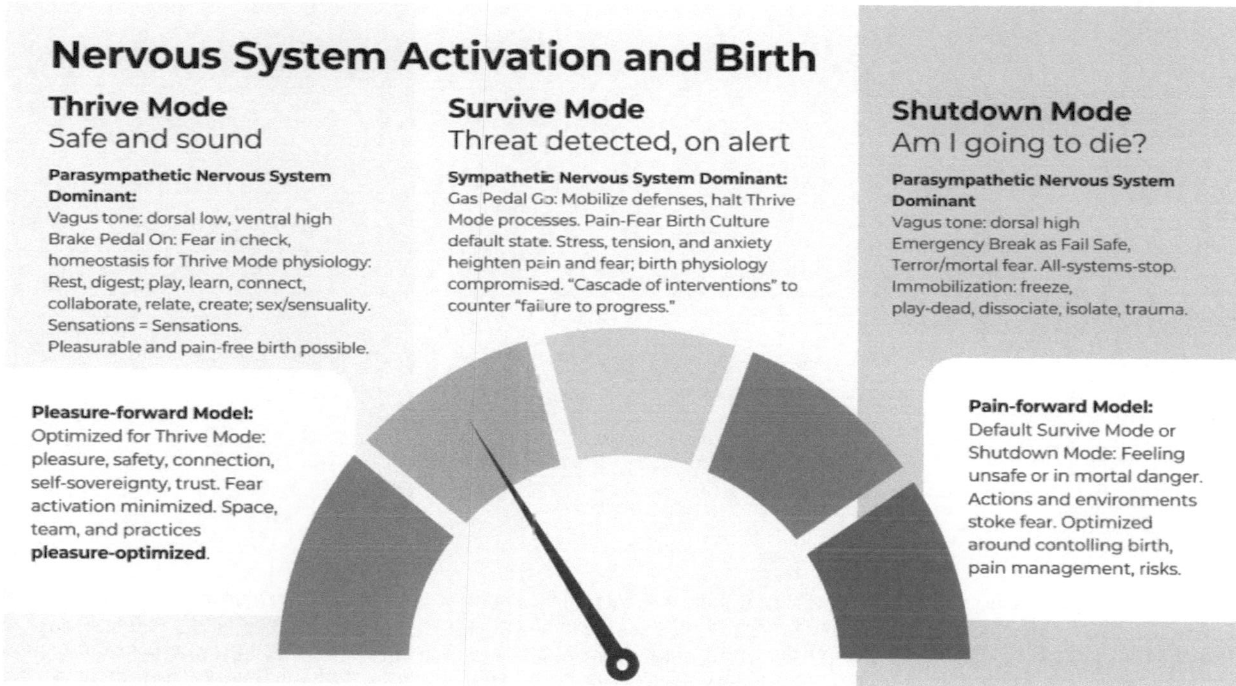

FIGURE 7.3 Application of the Pleasure-Forward Birth Model to Nervous System Activation Models.

Note. My development of this graphic had greatly been informed by multiple critical works of the following: American College of Nurse-Midwives (2013); Antonovsky (1987, 1996); Buckley (2002); Buckley and Dip (2003); Bolaza (2020); Beisecker (1990); Beck (2004); Basile (2012); Ballard et al. (1995); Creedy et al. (2000); Cho et al. (2013); Cahill (2001); Dana (2018); Dick-Read (1942/2004); Davis (2019); Davis-Floyd (1994, 2003, 2018, 2022), Davis and Pascali Bonaro (2010); Kitzinger (1997, 2011, 2013); Komisaruk (2016); Komisaruk and Whipple (1998, 2000); Komisaruk and Sansone (2003); Whipple and Komisaruk (1985, 1988); Whipple et al. (1990); Krieger & Fee (1994), Levin (1992, 2002, 2011); Lloyd (2005); MacDorman et al. (2016); Martin (2001); McCormack (2005); Melancon (2021); Meston and Frohlich (2000); Miller and Shriver (2012); Midwives Alliance of North America (2017); Neiterman (2013); Odent (1987; 1991, 2007, 2021); Oparah and Bonaparte (2015); Paltrow and Flavin (2013); Petchesky (1995); Porges (2018, 2022); Pranzarone (1991); Raymond (1993); Reyes-Lagos et al. (2019); Ross and Solinger (2017); Schlote (2021); Simkin (1991, 2006); SisterSong (2022); Slade (2000); Vedam et al., (2019); Wertz and Wertz (1989); Yeung and Pauls (2016).

and its sensations are experienced, and where relationality interfaces with the body (see Figure 7.2). *Head space* denotes the specific states of consciousness that had been reported in numerous interviews and apparently is essential for birth pleasure to unfold. It is in some ways a personal, mental, and emotional ambiance. In part it is also a mindset or an intentional orientation toward experiencing birth sensations without judgement, particularly sensations that typically are linked with fear, anxiety, or distress. In terms of polyvagal theory, this head space concept can be thought to help keep the birthing person within the sustainable Thrive Mode homeostatic physiology.

Relational Space

The next layer in The Pleasure-Forward Birth Model is the *relational space* around the birthing person, which includes the quality and quantity of this person's relationships and the active interactions that are occurring during the birth experience (Figure 7.1). To draw on polyvagal theory here, this relational space is where coregulation plays a powerful role, wherein the neurological mode of the birthing person can either be enhanced or disturbed by those around them in ways that operate beneath their conscious awareness. This relational space could be one to one (1:1), such as the intimacy between a birthing person and their partner or a doula. It could also be with many people whom the birthing person has chosen to support them during their birth (1:n), such as Venus's home birth during which some of her friends had soon arrived and had promptly headed to the kitchen to make a birthday cake, and the sound of joyful yet everyday conversation had played enhancing role within the relational space around her. It could also involve no one, in the case of one participant's hospital birth, during which their most pleasurable moments were found in solitude. Relational space may, depending on the birth setting and the birthing person, involve kinfolk, strangers, healthcare providers, neighbors, Uber drivers, clerical workers, passers-by, ancestors, and untold others.

Contextual Space

Wrapping around the relational space in the Pleasure-Forward Model of Birth is the *contextual space* of the setting in which a given birth takes place and the relationality around it. Simply put, the contextual space could be a hospital, an autonomous birth center, a home, or any other venue where birth occurs. Contextual space involves the birth ambiance and also involves the physical, natural, and built environments. It could also include the weather, the temperature, environmental exposures to toxins, and other contextual conditions that can be directly experienced during birth. Time is another critical aspect of the contextual space around the birthing people. The time of day, for example, is a major contextual factor impacting birth care, as is the day of the week, and even the season, most especially for hospital births because most US ob/gyns prefer not to work on the weekends, over holidays, nor in the late nights or early mornings (see Davis-Floyd, 2018, pp.107–140 and Davis-Floyd, 2022). There are also the features of birth setting, such as the policies, protocols, routines, norms, available resources and staffing, differing models of birth care and of birth management to consider at this level. For example, the contextual space is where a hospital policy that enables or bars labor support people of the birthing persons' choice, or that places rigid time limits on the various phases of labor, would be conceptualized in this model (again, see Figure 7.1).

Structural Space

In the Pleasure-Forward Birth Model, I use the term *structural space* to convey the larger political, legal, and institutional factors that in turn inform or shape the contextual and relational spaces (again, see Figure 7.1). For example, factors such as the private or public healthcare insurance involved in a specific birth care setting, or the number and capacities of care facilities within a given locality, such as rural or urban settings. Structural space also involves matters of access, resources, employment, income, transportation, and infrastructure. Politics, legislative statutes, legalities, policing, and bureaucracy that structure how the birthing person navigates their birth, and the contextual and relational impacts of those structures are also considered at the level of structural space. For example, health insurance covering/not covering doula or homebirth midwifery care and thereby empowering or foreclosing the option of choosing either would be conceptualized as part of the structural space. Also, the fact that we are currently seeing throughout the United States (predominantly in racialized, rural, and economically marginalized communities) closures of maternity wards and/or labor and delivery units in hospitals, or even entire hospitals, is a major structural-level concern.

Sociocultural Space

All these other spaces are permeated and surrounded by the *sociocultural space*, wherein paradigms, ideologies, cultural norms and beliefs, history, and other dynamic sociocultural forces such as racism, classism, sexism, cisheteronormativity, ableism, ageism, capitalism, militarism, and colonial and biomedical imperialism operate. The fact that maternal care closures are happening in disproportionately Black and Brown communities as well as predominantly White communities (particularly rural communities facing entrenched poverty) is a certainly sociocultural layer. I also think of liberation praxes, antiracism, myriad feminisms, decolonialism, and our relationship to the Earth on this level. So here, this is a level of liberatory praxis, where those of us who are concerned with transforming these injustices dream up new paradigms and futures, and take actions that may permeate through all the other layers of the Pleasure-Forward Birth Model (again, see Figure 7.1).

Applications of the Pleasure-Forward Birth Model

While reductionist and positivist modes of thinking about birth would be shallow and reprehensible in the face of these complex and nuanced data about birth, so too would be a model that is not useful or testable because it simply says: "everything affects everything." First, as I have often noted in the Introduction to this book and in many of its preceding chapters that this study had been a mixed-methods one that I had grounded first and foremost in the qualitative ethnographic work that I have featured throughout this book: a study that I had specifically designed to explore a formerly mostly unstudied topic, and not to rigorously test hypotheses. By having conducted this study, I had aimed to provide some foundational investigation of its own merit, but on which further such studies must be developed. But for now, I want to provide an actionable tool that is based on the rich findings that I have presented herein. I have developed an Orientation Tool (Figure 7.4) to offer a practical framework for birthing people and to those who care for them to think through their own orientations toward births and to evaluate the alignment of those who are inside of their r*elational space*, whether passive or active, toward birth pleasure. So doing can help them to identify actionable factors to consider in each quadrant depending on the unique circumstances, resources, barriers, and risk factors as relevant to a particular birthing person within their multiple contexts as I've described just above.

The study participants fell into two camps. First, there were those who had an active orientation toward birth pleasure, for example, Bree and Calisto actively sought and cultivated their experiences of birth pleasure through preparation and intentional birth team building. Then there were those who'd done nothing of the sort. Some had a passive orientation toward birth pleasure because they'd been unaware that it was possible. And yet, their experiences had been pleasurable in whole or in part, for example, Chandra's pain-free birth or Dalisay's mystical experiences at

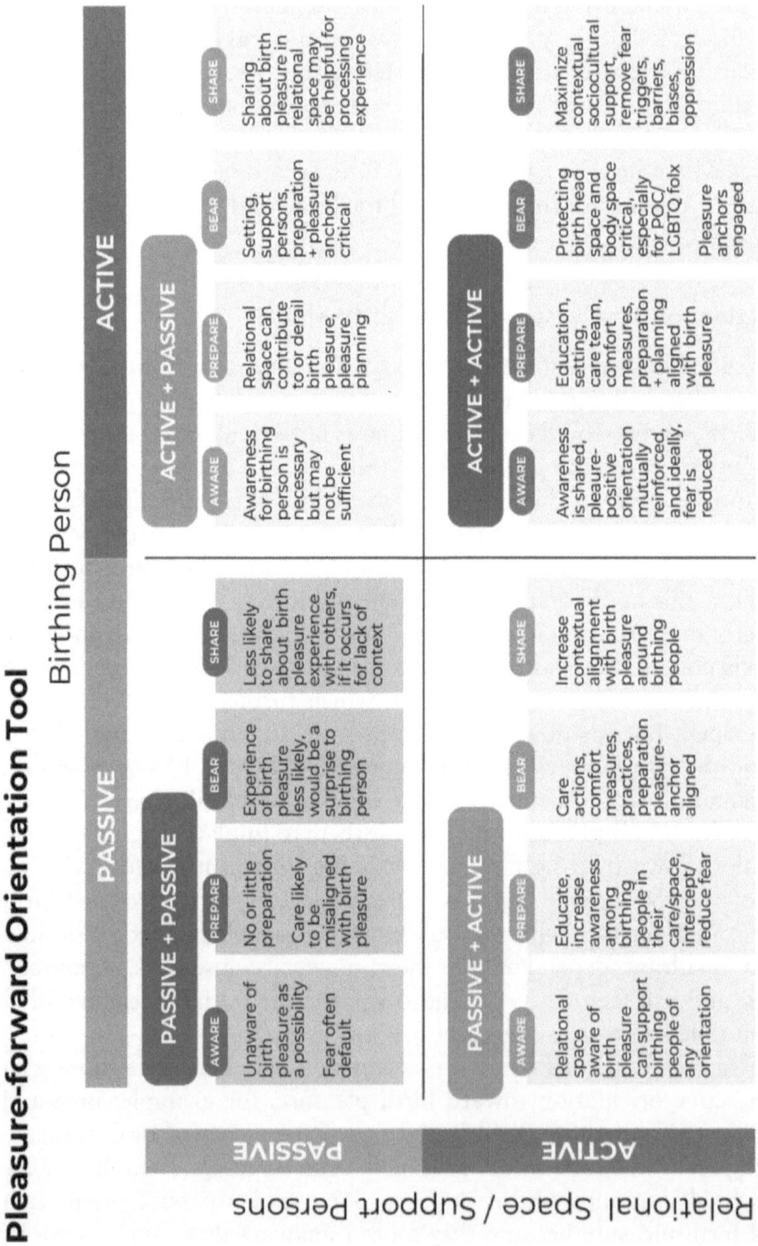

FIGURE 7.4 Pleasure-Forward Model Orientation Tool.

delivery. (Again, see Chapter 6.) Other participants had fully been aware of the possibility of experiencing pleasure but had not thought that it would happen to them, like Romi. I would say that Marion's orientation toward birth pleasure shifted from passive to active from her first to her second birth. Similarly, Araceli dismissed hypnobirth during her first pregnancy, viewing the approach as "silly" and "woo-woo," but later, she reconsidered, and fully embraced the method during her second pregnancy, and with great success. For the passive orientation group, their experiences of birth pleasure were unanticipated and surprising, about which they'd typically been reluctant to share with anyone else for the reasons that I have explained above and in preceding chapters. Then, there'd been the matter of the immediate relational environment, or their relational space of partners, care providers, kin, friends, acquaintances, and others, and their passive or active orientations toward birth pleasure. There might have also been antagonistic orientations toward birth pleasure, which had not been mentioned during these interviews but which would deserve a rigorous scholarly analysis. I hope that those who have an active orientation toward birth pleasure will not have to contend with antagonism around them, but this antagonism is foreseeable given the current state of birth culture in the US and elsewhere. This tool offers starting points for both identifying and for reconciling the multiple discordances in birthing peoples' orientations toward pleasure in birth—starting from the center of the Pleasure-Forward Birth Model (the birthing person) as compared with those around them (relational). A similar approach could assist in the analyses of their immediate birth environment (contextual), the factors shaping this environment, such as hospital policies (structural), and perhaps ultimately the sociocultural factors that permeate the other layers of the Model.

As previously noted, and to recap here, birth pleasure may be a symptom of birth wellbeing, a salutogenic signal that reinforces healthy birth physiology. In contrast, the "cascade of interventions" is a term used by many childbirth educators and birth activists for problematic and routine overuse of medical interventions in birth, which in a vicious cycle build on each other and toward increased odds of cesareans that might have otherwise been avoidable (Tracy et al., 2007). In this Pleasure-Forward Birth Model, I propose that, in a virtuous cycle, a cascade of elations, indeed of pleasurable experiences, might build toward heightened birth wellbeing. It can't hurt, can it? Of course, none of my study participants reported any harms from the pleasurable aspects of their birth experiences, but there is surely more research that needs to be done in this arena.

Access to positive, pleasurable experiences, and arguably salutary factors, protective factors, and the removal of obstacles and barriers are predictably patterned by social and structural determinants of health.

These determinants can be understood as interacting layers, as in the bioecological systems model that centers on the individual level and then expands in reflexive causality, varying with the birth paradigm and the model of care at play for any particular birthing person, their birth setting, and context. Here, I present a quote from one study participant, Chandra, who viewed the cultural challenges at hand in crystalline clarity:

> Birth is only challenging because the environment that we live in is artificial and challenging. There's nothing human about how we live, civilization has nothing to do with being a human being. Nothing. And that's why we suffer. It, again, in my opinion, and all of our issues—mental health issues and physical health issues and birthing baby issues and poor parenting, mating, marrying, is all happening because it's being done in this artificial construct. And people feel bad about themselves, or they feel like they're losers when they feel they can't do it. And I want to tell people that it's not you. It's the environment around you. And we're supposed to be able to do something as elemental as reproduction. Reproduction is elemental. A bedbug can do it. Your kitty can do it. Why can't you—smart human that can do algebra?

Chandra's question is legitimate. Indeed, why can't we? In Chapter 1, I sketched out how we got to this point, and the many stories that I've shared in this book illustrate much about the impacts of this history and suggest new ways forward. Changing any aspect of the hegemonic birth culture or its drivers (the structural and social determinants externally, and then perhaps internalized within birthing bodies through psychological and neurological processes such as coregulation), could involve praxis—a critical pedagogical cycle of action and reflection toward justice articulated by radical educator Paulo Freire (1970). For birth culture to shift away from a pain/fear/risk model to something more expansive and inclusive of pleasure and wellbeing, the application of this Pleasure-Forward Birth Model will have to expand beyond the individual birthing person's experiences. Most of my interview participants, at least those who had not been completely blindsided by birth pleasure, followed a pattern of evolution into and through a pleasurable birth experience. They started out unaware of pleasurable (or pain-free) birth as a possibility, then, had somehow become aware, next they had chosen to prepare, and then to bear the experience of birth pleasure-forward and/or pain-free from this orientation. Many of these participants had wanted to share about their pleasurable experiences with others, a desire which was not always acted upon but would have contributed to others becoming aware that pain and fear are not the only ways in which birth can be experienced. Their stories

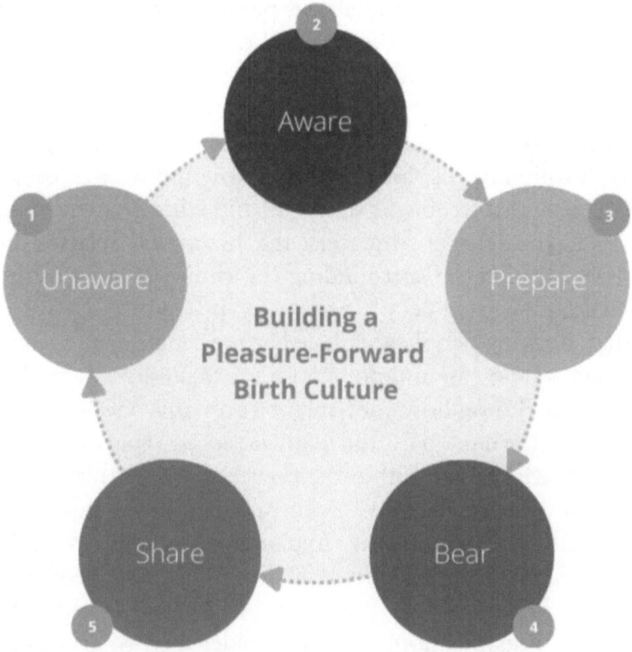

FIGURE 7.5 Praxis Model.

had sketched out a simple praxis model of building a pleasure-forward birth culture by, for, and with birthing people (see Figure 7.5). There is no doubt that these praxis processes are impinged upon or are enhanced by the myriads of social and structural forces at play. Any one of these aspects of this praxis cycle could contribute to the creation of a pleasure-forward birth culture. Surely, this book is a part of this praxis because this book has been written by a birthing person who is unapologetically working hard to shift birth culture toward something more just and wonderful, through research and education.

In contrast to typical academic health research, this study is not intended only for academics, physicians, nor for other professional healthcare authorities. First and foremost, this study and the Model that has emerged from it is by and for birthing people. Second, it is for all those who serve birthing people. Through this Pleasure-Forward Model I intend to challenge the hegemonic hierarchy in birth-related knowledge production by shifting the presumed audience for such knowledge and thereby the impact of this Model. This Model is also different in that it accommodates multiple birth care modalities, care settings, levels of medicalization, and social contexts because it decenters highly medicalized hospital birth as the default. It also decenters the biomedical model's pathogenesis paradigm to accommodate pleasure and salutogenesis (which is the study of the origins of health that focuses on factors that support human wellbeing, rather than on factors that cause disease/pathogenesis). It does *not* define birth as a medical condition nor treat biomedical care as the only model available to birthing people. It makes room for hospital births, for births in autonomous birth centers, home births, and unattended freebirths wherever and whenever they might occur. This Model also attempts to discern the functional relationships between the spheres of influence surrounding (by choice or not) birthing people, without making birthing people passive recipients of those spheres of influence. Rather, birthing people are placed at the center as the seats of power, as whole beings who can and do choose for themselves what birth is and is not. They can choose how they might apply this Model to their navigation of birth. For the most part, the many layers or "spaces" that are articulated within this Model are within the power of the birthing person to choose, adjust, or decline. However, the application of this Model must never descend into rote, prescriptive application. By addressing their orientations toward each space (as suits their lives), birthing people and those who serve them can ensure this Model is, as it was designed, a tool for empowerment and humanization. Next, I consider the two groups that I most want to reach with these findings: birthing people and birth justice advocates/activists.

Birth justice has been described as a vision that: "every pregnant person should have an empowering birthing experience, free of unnecessary medical interventions and forced separation from their child" (Black Women Birthing Justice [BWBJ], 2023). A more commonly used term, *reproductive justice*, has been defined as "the human right to maintain personal bodily autonomy, have children, not have children, and parent the children we have in safe and sustainable communities" (Asian Communities for Reproductive Justice, 2023; SisterSong, 2022). It should be noted that this definition of reproductive justice does not address birth itself. Silliman et al. (2004) highlighted movements for reproductive rights and reproductive justice led by Women of Color who have and continue to disproportionately experience and challenge reproductive oppression. Many birth justice advocates have argued that birth itself must be included for reproductive justice to be fully realized (Diaz-Tello & Paltrow, 2010; Oparah & BWBJ, 2016). Also led by Women of Color, birth justice activism has grown as a movement, roughly during the early 2010s, to address the intersecting oppressions facing women and birthing People of Color, to challenge the racist, classist, and cisheteronormative frames that remain pervasive within the natural birth and homebirth midwifery movements (Cheyney, 2008; Craven, 2010). Yet, since these publications, birth movements have become more inclusive over time as their multiple proponents have gained greater awareness of these important issues (see, for examples, Davis & Craven, 2022) and have come to view birth as a nexus of both social justice transformation and empowerment (Oparah & BWBJ, 2016).

Implications and Recommendations

A multidimensional understanding of birth pleasure will better serve birthing people, recognizing them as complex human beings who are moving through a life-changing process. The *Pleasure-Forward Birth Model*, and perhaps such a birth culture, I argue, should be a part of this expanded understanding. What are the implications of this study for those who are most interested in birth wellbeing? What can I recommend to them based on the findings of my research? I start where I believe all birth research should start: with birthing people.

Birthing People

> Your body's yours. Your birth is yours!
>
> *(Fabia)*

It is beyond question that birthing people themselves have the most to gain and lose in giving birth. Their birth experiences will impact them, for better or worse, for the rest of their lives. Their very lives are on the line, and they know it. The key application of my study's findings, as I see it, is for a wide expansion of the existing social scripts about birth in three key directions. First, it must extend far beyond the current fear-pain frame to a much more expansive one that makes enough space for a broad array of both pleasurable and challenging experiences during birth: a pleasure-positive point of view or *mindset*. Second, the study participants had collectively created a container for their birthing: *head space*. Third, they had fully demonstrated an intentionality about pleasure by having consciously used what I call: *pleasure anchors*. Fourth, they had completely dismantled the ignorant-patient/omniscient-care-provider dichotomy from their own perspectives, to *center themselves* as being the most important in the birthing space. The ability to center themselves is entwined with the choice of birth *setting*, which is crucial. These factors stand out as focal points that birthing people can apply to their birth preparation. I am certainly not the first to call attention to these ideas. My findings both echo and substantiate similar calls by many birth justice and birth wellbeing advocates, care providers, and educators across decades of US birth politics. Much of what

I synthesize below are things that these study participants had shared with me during our lengthy and in-depth interviews in hopes that others might learn from their experiences.

Birthing people have many choices to make leading up to their births. The data in this study iterate some key factors that rest within the power of birthing people. First is their *mindset* toward their births. My study participants did not tend to view birth as fundamentally painful or terrifying. They chose to view the birth process in a way that left them feeling safe, empowered, and joyful. This was particularly true among those who gave birth pain-free without anesthesia. They chose to experience the birth process as sensations of pressure, stretching, and even pleasure, as opposed to deciding in advance that whatever they felt was pain. They also engaged in practices that empowered a pleasure-forward point of view and intentionally steered clear of people, spaces, and structures that disrupted their pleasurable birthing experiences. They were adamant that they were not special "unicorns" as Melissa put it—that their birth experiences were the result of intentional practices available to most anyone and not a matter of dumb luck. There is much work that needs to be done to shift the cultural consciousness around birth itself. Birthing people and those who serve them must unlearn the normative sociocultural scripts that have done tremendous harm, and create new ones that do the opposite—enhance and uplift wellbeing.

Protecting the special birthing *head space* emerged as paramount over and over in my research. There are many ways that this can be done. Some of my study participants used hypnobirthing techniques to train themselves. Some used other birth preparation courses or practices such as prenatal yoga and meditation. But all involved the choice to fully own the experience, view birth afresh, consistently reinforce that new perspective, and protect their *head space* from disruptions. Folks with histories of trauma, racialized abuse, or violence had work to do to create safety around themselves so that they could truly be with their birthing experience and maintain that special *head space*. Some crafted rituals and wrapped themselves in caring support teams and trusted loved ones. Some sought solitude. All sought a place both within and outside of their birthing bodies that made them feel good. Pleasure requires honesty with oneself and others to emerge.

Third, *pleasure anchors* were central to many of the birth experiences shared in this book. Again, I note that emotional pleasure seems to be the first, most foundational layer of birth pleasure. Anything that supported relaxation or triggered gladness and gratitude facilitated the birth process. Almost all of the pleasurable experiences that I've captured herein involved some sense of gladness for birth process—excitement, anticipation, joy, gratitude, and even relief. For some, *pleasure anchors* were the caresses of their partner, breathing together, a kiss on the forehead, or the removal of negative stimuli, the calming feel of cool tile to the forehead, to the subtle ways light and music gave pleasure, to clitoral stimulation. For some birthing people, it will require an investigation to discover what creates pleasure, and the courage to use what they discover works for them. A degree of intentionality about pleasure and an openness to the birth experience were present in many of these interviews. While none of the participants articulated it in these terms, I would love to see birthing people developing "pleasure management plans" as they often do for their "pain management plans" as a large part of their birth planning and team building.

Fourth, my participants iterated in several ways that the choice of care *setting* is paramount to their ability to *center themselves* within the birth experience. Setting greatly correlates with the style of care that is received and with whom. Context matters, and a good match between a birthing person's desired care style and their choice of birth setting goes a long way in laying the groundwork for a pleasurable birth experience. This study has clearly illustrated that hospital births and highly medicalized styles of care were less likely to be pleasurable. This finding echoed across the interviews, wherein unsatisfying births had tended to involve care providers with a view of many of their patients as ignorant, and their own knowledge as infallible and total. Wherever this dichotomy dominated, birthing people suffered. Birthing people must first see themselves as the authorities of their own bodily experiences and should demand that their knowledge be treated with the credence that it deserves. They must not accept care providers who diminish or dismiss their own embodied and intellectual knowledge. Care providers can view the birthing person's knowledge as being either authoritative or subordinate. What study participants who had experienced birth pleasure communicated overall in these data is that the most important person in the birthing room should always be the birthing person. This runs counter to the culturally normative social scripts that tend to choreograph care interactions from a default state of ignorance on the part of the patient and centrality and omniscience on the part of the care providers. Neither is total. This kind of hierarchical, binary thinking must be dismantled for more nuanced, real, collaborative, and just care relationships to thrive.

Birth Justice Advocates and Activists

Birth spaces are far too often sites of oppression, violation, trauma, suffering, illness, and death, particularly for Black, Brown, and Indigenous birthing people (see Liese et al., 2021). Birth justice advocates and activists are struggling against these institutional and societal constructions of birth that have resulted in birth environments and care paradigms that often sabotage birth wellbeing, as Aleks put it: "systems designed to make you fail at birth." They are also in the game of creating something else, something better. Birth pleasure might well become an aspect of this creation. As brown (2019; a doula) in *Pleasure Activism* has suggested, pleasure is a compass by which we might find a path toward justice, and while pain is deeply instructive, so too is pleasure. This study offers, humbly, an expanded view of the birth experience, not to derail a conversation about the injustices and suffering faced by birthing people. By addressing pleasure too, my intention is to humanize the birthing person as capable of more than just enduring pain and evading danger, but also of relishing in enjoyment, delight, and ecstasy in birth. For birth justice advocates and activists, this study both points toward and highlights the ways in which birth pleasure arises in defiance in the ingenuity and genius of those navigating oppressive, racist, classist, cisheteronormative, ableist birth environments, and their victories. It is an ode to their joy, courage, and generosity to share this with others, in the hope that their experiences might make someone else's journey lighter and make them feel better. Engaging with pleasure can be a personal political project as well as an interpersonal or a sociocultural one. All have their relative levers for worldmaking.

Within the individual activist, having a solid relationship with pleasure as a personal resource and guiding compass might help to empower new kinds of activism and relationship-building for a future of justice in birth. There may be healing work to do in this regard, particularly for those who have suffered birth trauma themselves and vicariously through others. This healing work is activism. Healing will involve methods that are as unique as those people who pursue it. Creating safe spaces for this healing and for the reclamation of pleasure in community may help activists move in the direction of pleasure, and perhaps, then, spread a pleasure-forward perspective out from there: as within, so without.

Many birth justice activists are birthworkers deeply involved in the care of birthing people. If birth pleasure is not yet a part of their paradigm, perhaps this study will be an opportunity to expand in this direction, with an evidence base to substantiate both innovative and ancestral approaches to birthwork. The suggestions that I've made to birth care providers above might be applicable starting places, but just as likely are traditional knowledges that pre-date biomedical imperialism and connect birthing people across time and space. The concepts that I've included in this book, such as fostering a Pleasure-Forward point of view of birth, discussing pleasure management, having a pleasure plan, discovering, practicing, and using pleasure anchors might be helpful to birthing people.

I ask birthworkers of all disciplines to consider using the Pleasure-Forward Birth Model presented herein, and the Pleasure-Forward Birth Orientation Tool with clients or other practitioners.

Birth justice activists also engage with care settings that are unsupportive or are actively hostile to their work and are thereby inhibitory of birth pleasure. I suggest that such activists might organize with respected colleagues, collaborate with birthing people and birthworkers, and develop methods of expanding awareness of birth pleasure as a possibility worthy of support. This awareness could be achieved through midwifery and doula practices, childbirth educator practices, new parent/mother groups, online spaces, organizations, and more. The informal networks of care that help birthing people navigate their paths toward birth can play a huge role here. The people who participate in these networks can share information about what location-specific spaces, care providers, and institutions are more supportive of birth pleasure approaches than others. Based on this study's findings, I can suggest that some birthing people might consider home birth to better ensure that their birth approaches are respected and that their desired pleasure measures can be employed freely and without shame or fear.

Ultimately, accountability for injustice and harms in birth spaces might be the long fight. The pursuit of positive and pleasurable birth is an immediate opportunity. The Birth Pleasure Study has, for me, been both a praxis and an act of love for those of us who give birth—who make the world anew from within their own depths. May birthgiving—bringing new lives into being—be deeply recognized as the profound act of worldmaking that it is, as an exquisite rebellion against oppression, and as a wild celebration of the chance we each get to be alive.

References

American College of Nurse-Midwives. (2013). Supporting healthy and normal physiologic childbirth: A consensus statement by ACNM, MANA, and NACPM. *Journal of Perinatal Education*, *22*(1), 14–18. https://doi.org/10.1891/1058-1243.22.1.14

Antonovsky, A. (1987). *Unraveling the mystery of health*. Jossey-Bass.

Antonovsky, A. (1996). The salutogenic model as a theory to guide health promotion. *Health Promotion International*, *11*(1), 11–18. https://doi.org/10.1093/heapro/11.1.11

Asian Communities for Reproductive Justice. (2023). *Reproductive justice agenda*. https://apirh.org/reproductive.html

Balban, M. Y., Neri, E., Kogon, M. M., Weed, L., Nouriani, B., Jo, B., ... & Huberman, A. D. (2023). Brief structured respiration practices enhance mood and reduce physiological arousal. *Cell Reports Medicine*, *4*(1) 1–10; e1–e4.

Ballard, C., Stanley, K., & Brockington, I. (1995). Post-traumatic stress disorder after childbirth. *British Journal of Psychiatry*, *166*(4), 525–528. https://doi.org/10.1192/bjp.166.4.525

Basile, M. R. (2012). *Reproductive justice and childbirth reform: Doulas as agents of social change* [Doctoral dissertation, The University of Iowa]. The University of Iowa's Institutional Repository.

Bauer, G. F, & Jenny, G. J. (2007). Development, implementation and dissemination of Occupational Health Management (OHM): Putting salutogenesis into practice. In S. McIntyre & J. Houdmont (Eds.), *Occupational health psychology: European perspectives on research, education and practice* (Vol. 2, pp. 219–250). ISMAI.

Beck, C. T. (2004). Birth trauma: In the eye of the beholder. *Nursing Research*, *53*(1), 28–35. https://doi.org/10.1097/00006199-200401000-00005

Beisecker, A. E. (1990). Patient power in doctor–patient communication: What do we know?. *Health Communication*, *2*(2), 105–122. https://doi.org/10.1207/s15327027hc0202_4

Black Women Birthing Justice. (2023). *Birth justice*. www.blackwomenbirthingjustice.com/birth-justice

Bolaza, E. B. (2020). Birth pleasure: Meanings, politics, and praxis. *Journal of the Motherhood Initiative for Research and Community Involvement*, *11*(1) 123–135. https://jarm.journals.yorku.ca/index.php/jarm/article/view/40595

Bolton, D., Gillett, G., Bolton, D., & Gillett, G. (2019). The biopsychosocial model 40 years on. *The Biopsychosocial Model of Health and Disease: New Philosophical and Scientific Developments*, 1–43. https://doi.org/10.1007/978-3-030-11899-0_1

Bronfenbrenner, U. (1974). Developmental research, public policy, and the ecology of childhood. *Child Development*, *45*(1), 1–5. https://doi.org/10.2307/1127743

Bronfenbrenner, U. (1977). Toward an experimental ecology of human development. *American Psychologist*, *32*(7), 513. https://psycnet.apa.org/doi/10.1037/0003-066X.32.7.513

Bronfenbrenner, U., & Ceci, S. J. (1994). Nature–nurture reconceptualized in developmental perspective: A bioecological model. *Psychological Review*, *101*(4), 568–586. https://doi.org/10.1037/0033-295X.101.4.568

Brown, A. M. (2019). *Pleasure activism: The politics of feeling good*. AK Press.

Buckley, S. J. (2002). Ecstatic birth: The hormonal blueprint of labor. *Mothering Magazine*, *111*, 59–68. www.mothering.com/threads/ecstatic-birth.1622545/

Buckley, S. J., & Dip, O. (2003, Summer). Undisturbed birth: Nature's blueprint for ease and ecstasy. *Journal of Prenatal and Perinatal Psychology and Health*, *17*, 261–288. www.birthpsychology.com/wp-content/uploads/journal/published_paper/volume-17/issue-4/06xgsNya.pdf

Cahill, H. A. (2001), Male appropriation and medicalization of childbirth: An historical analysis. *Journal of Advanced Nursing*, *33*, 334–342. https://doi.org/10.1046/j.1365-2648.2001.01669.x

Cheyney, M. J. (2008). Homebirth as systems-challenging praxis: Knowledge, power, and intimacy in the birthplace. *Qualitative Health Research*, *18*(2), 254–267. https://doi.org/10.1177/1049732307312393

Cho, S., Crenshaw, K. W., & McCall, L. (2013). Toward a field of intersectionality studies: Theory, applications, and praxis. *Signs: Journal of Women in Culture and Society*, *38*(4), 785–810. https://doi.org/10.1086/669608

Choi, J. M., Padmala, S., Spechler, P., & Pessoa, L. (2014). Pervasive competition between threat and reward in the brain. *Social Cognitive and Affective Neuroscience*, *9*(6), 737–750. https://doi.org/10.1093/scan/nst053

Craven, C. (2010). *Pushing for midwives: Homebirth mothers and the reproductive rights movement*. Temple University Press.

Creedy, D. K., Shochet, I. M., & Horsfall, J. (2000). Childbirth and the development of acute trauma symptoms: Incidence and contributing factors. *Birth*, 27(2), 104–111. https://doi.org/10.1046/j.1523-536x.2000.00104.x

Crossing, P. (2021). Pain and pleasure in the birthing room: Understanding the phenomenon of orgasmic birth. *British Journal of Midwifery*, *29*(8), 464–471. https://doi.org/10.12968/bjom.2021.29.8.464

Dana, D. (2018). *The polyvagal theory in therapy: Engaging the rhythm of regulation (Norton series on interpersonal neurobiology)*. W. W. Norton.

Davis, D. A. (2019). Obstetric racism: The racial politics of pregnancy, labor, and birthing. *Medical Anthropology*, *38*(7), 560–573. https://doi.org/10.1080/01459740.2018.1549389

Davis, E., & Pascali Bonaro, D. (2010). *Orgasmic birth: Your guide to a safe, satisfying, and pleasurable birth experience*. Rodale.

Davis-Floyd, R. (1994). The technocratic body: American childbirth as cultural expression. *Social Science & Medicine*, *38*(8), 1125–1140. https://doi.org/10.1016/0277-9536(94)90228-3

Davis-Floyd, R. (2003). *Birth as an American rite of passage: With a new preface*. University of California Press.

Davis-Floyd, R. (2018). *Ways of knowing about birth: Mothers, midwives, medicine, and birth activism*. Waveland Press.

Davis-Floyd, R. (2022). *Birth as an American rite of passage* (3rd ed.). Routledge.

Dick-Read, G. (2004). Childbirth without fear: The principles and practice of natural childbirth. Pinter & Martin. (Original work published 1942).

Engel, G. L. (1978). The biopsychosocial model and the education of health professionals. *Annals of the New York Academy of Sciences*, *310*(1), 169–181. https://doi.org/10.1016/0163-8343(79)90062-8

Freire, P. (1970). Pedagogy of the oppressed (M. Bergman Ramos, Trans.). Continuum.

Kitzinger, S. (1997). *Authoritative touch in childbirth: A cross-cultural approach*. University of California Press.

Kitzinger, S. (2011). *Rediscovering birth*. Pinter & Martin.

Kitzinger, S. (2013). *Birth & sex: The power and the passion*. Pinter & Martin.

Komisaruk, B. R. (2016). Commentary on "The Evolutionary Origin of Female Orgasm" by M. Pavličev and G. Wagner, 2016. *Journal of Experimental Zoology Part B: Molecular and Developmental Evolution*, *326*(8), 504–506. https://doi.org/10.1002/jez.b.22712

Komisaruk, B. R., & Sansone, G. (2003). Neural pathways mediating vaginal function: The vagus nerves and spinal cord oxytocin. *Scandinavian Journal of Psychology*, *44*(3), 241–250. https://doi.org/10.1111/1467-9450.00341

Komisaruk, B. R., & Whipple, B. (1998). Love as sensory stimulation: Physiological consequences of its deprivation and expression. *Psychoneuroendocrinology*, *23*, 927–944. https://doi.org/10.1016/S0306-4530(98)00062-6

Komisaruk, B. R., & Whipple, B. (2000). How does vaginal stimulation produce pleasure, pain, and analgesia? In R. B. Fillingim (Ed.), *Sex, gender, and pain* (pp. 109–134). IASP Press.

Krieger, N., & Fee, E. (Eds.). (1994). *Women's health, politics, and power*. Routledge. https://doi.org/10.4324/9781315231020

Levin, R. J. (1992). The mechanisms of human female sexual arousal. *Annual Review of Sex Research*, *3*(1), 1–48. https://doi.org/10.1080/10532528.1992.10559874

Levin, R. J. (2002). The physiology of sexual arousal in the human female: A recreational and procreational synthesis. *Archives of Sexual Behavior*, *31*(5), 405–411. https://doi.org/10.1023/A:1019836007416

Levin, R. J. (2011, June). Can the controversy about the putative role of the human female orgasm in sperm transport be settled with our current physiological knowledge of coitus? *Journal of Sexual Medicine*, *8*(6), 1566–1578. https://doi.org/10.1111/j.1743-6109.2010.02162.x

Liese K., Davis-Floyd R., Stewart K., & Cheyney, M. (2021). Obstetric iatrogenesis in the United States: The spectrum of unintentional harm, disrespect, violence, and abuse. *Anthropology & Medicine* *28*(2), 188–204. https://doi.org/10.1080/13648470.2021.1938510

Lloyd, E. A. (2005). *The case of the female orgasm: Bias in the science of evolution*. Harvard University Press.

MacDorman, M. F., Declercq, E., Cabral, H., & Morton, C. (2016). Is the United States maternal mortality rate increasing? Disentangling trends from measurement issues. *Obstetrics and Gynecology*, *128*(3), 447–455. http://doi.org/10.1097/AOG.0000000000001556.

Martin, E. (2001). *The woman in the body: A cultural analysis of reproduction*. Beacon Press.

McCormack, K. (2005). Stratified reproduction and poor women's resistance. *Gender & Society*, *19*(5), 660–679. https://doi.org/10.1177/0891243205278010

Melancon, S. (2021). Safety, co-regulation, and polyvagal theory: The autonomic nervous system as the missing link in childbirth outcomes and experiences. In R. Davis-Floyd (Ed.), *Birthing techno-sapiens: Human-technology co-evolution and the future of reproduction* (pp. 208–221). Routledge.

Meston, C. M., & Frohlich, P. F. (2000). The neurobiology of sexual function. *Archives of General Psychiatry*, *57*(11), 1012–1030. https://psycnet.apa.org/doi/10.1001/archpsyc.57.11.1012

Midwives Alliance of North America. (2017). *Statement of values and ethics*. MANA Core Documents. https://mana.org/resources/statement-of-values-and-ethics.

Miller, A. C., & Shriver, T. E. (2012). Women's childbirth preferences and practices in the United States. *Social Science & Medicine*, *75*(4), 709–716. https://doi.org/10.1016/j.socscimed.2012.03.051

Neiterman E. (2013). Sharing bodies: The impact of the biomedical model of pregnancy on women's embodied experiences of the transition to motherhood.

Healthcare Policy, *9*(Special Issue), 112–125. PMCID: PMC4750156. https://doi.org/10.12927/hcpol.2013.23595

Odent, M. (1987). The fetus ejection reflex. *Birth: Issues in Perinatal Care*, *14*(2), 104–105. https://doi.org/10.1111/j.1523-536X.1987.tb01463.x

Odent, M. (1991). Fear of death during labour. *Journal of Reproductive and Infant Psychology*, *9*(1), 43–47. https://doi.org/10.1080/02646839108403655

Odent, M. (2007). *Birth and breastfeeding: Rediscovering the needs of women during pregnancy and childbirth*. Clairview Books.

Odent, M. (2021). Is labor a complication of socialized birth? *Midwifery Today*. www.midwiferytoday.com/mt-articles/is-labor-a-complication-of-socialized-birth/

Oparah, J. C., & Bonaparte, A. D. (Eds.). (2015). *Birthing justice: Black women, pregnancy, and childbirth*. Routledge.

Oparah, J. C., & Black Women Birthing Justice. (2016). Beyond coersion and malign neglect: Black women and the struggle for birth justice, Introduction. In J. C. Oparah & A. D. Bonaparte (Eds.), *Birthing justice: Black women, pregnancy, and childbirth*. Routledge.

Paltrow, L. M., & Flavin, J. (2013). Arrests of and forced interventions on pregnant women in the United States, 1973–2005: Implications for women's legal status and public health. *Journal of Health Politics, Policy and Law*, *38*(2), 299–343. https://doi.org/10.1215/03616878-1966324

Petchesky, R. P. (1995). The body as property: A feminist re-vision. In F. D. Ginsburg & R. Rapp (Eds.), *Conceiving the new world order: The global politics of reproduction* (pp. 387–406). University of California Press.

Porges, S. W. (2009). The polyvagal theory: New insights into adaptive reactions of the autonomic nervous system. *Cleveland Clinic Journal of Medicine*, *76*(Suppl 2), S86. https://doi.org/10.3949%2Fccjm.76.s2.17

Porges, S. W. (2018). Polyvagal theory: A primer. In S. W. Porges & D. Dana (Eds.), *Clinical applications of the polyvagal theory: The emergence of polyvagal-informed therapies* (pp. 50–69). W. W. Norton.

Porges, S. W. (2022). Polyvagal theory: A science of safety. *Frontiers in Integrative Neuroscience*, *16*, 27. https://doi.org/10.3389/fnint.2022.871227

Pranzarone, G. F. (1991). Sexuoerotic stimulation and orgasmic response in the induction and management of parturition—clinical possibilities. In P. Kothari & R. Patel (Eds.), *Proceedings of First International Conference on Orgasm* (pp. 105–119). VRP.

Raymond, J. G. (1993). *Women as wombs: Reproductive technologies and the battle over women's freedom*. Spinifex Press.

Reyes-Lagos, J. J., Ledesma-Ramírez, C. I., Pliego-Carrillo, A. C., Peña-Castillo, M. Á., Echeverría, J. C., Becerril-Villanueva, E., Pavón, L., & Pacheco-López, G. (2019). Neuroautonomic activity evidences parturition as a complex and integrated neuro–immune–endocrine process. *Annals of the New York Academy of Sciences*, *1437*(1), 22–30. https://doi.org/10.1111/nyas.13860

Roach, J. (2020). ROOTT's theoretical framework of the web of causation between structural and social determinants of health and wellness—2016. *Restoring Our Own Through Transformation (ROOTT)*. www.roottrj.org/web-causation

Ross, L., & Solinger, R. (2017). *Reproductive justice: An introduction*. University of California Press.

Sandall, J., Soltani, H., Gates, S., Shennan, A., & Devane, D. (2013). Midwife-led continuity models versus other models of care for childbearing women. *Cochrane Database of Systematic Review*, *8*(8), 1–91. https://doi.org/10.1002/14651858.CD004667.pub5

Schlote, S. (2021). The polyvagal defense hierarchy. [Infographic]. The polyvagal theory and horses: An introduction. *EQUUSOMA*. https://equusoma.com/the-polyvagal-theory-and-horses/

Simkin, P. (1991). Just another day in a woman's life? Women's long-term perceptions of their first birth experience. Part I. *Birth*, *18*(4), 203–210. https://doi.org/10.1111/j.1523-536X.1991.tb00103.x

Simkin, P. (2006). What makes a good birth and why does it matter? *International Journal of Childbirth Education*, *21*(3), 4–6.

Silliman, J., Ross, L., Gutiérrez, E., & Gerber, M. (2004). *Undivided rights: Women of color organizing for reproductive justice*. Haymarket Books.

SisterSong. (2022). *Reproductive justice*. www.sistersong.net/reproductive-justice

Slade, P. (2000). Prevalence and predictors of posttraumatic stress symptoms following childbirth. *British Journal of Clinical Psychology*, *39*, 35–51. https://doi.org/10.1348/014466500163095

Tracy, S. K., Sullivan, E., Wang, Y. A., Black, D., & Tracy, M. (2007). Birth outcomes associated with interventions in labour amongst low risk women: A population-based study. *Women and Birth*, *20*(2), 41–48. https://doi.org/10.1016/j.wombi.2007.03.005

Vedam, S., Stoll, K., Taiwo, T. K., Rubashkin, N., Cheyney, M., Strauss, N., McLemore, M., Cadena, M., Nethery, E., Rushton, E., Schummers, L., Declercq, E., & the GVtM-US Steering Council. (2019). The Giving Voice to Mothers study: Inequity and mistreatment during pregnancy and childbirth in the United States. *Reproductive Health*, *16*(1), 1–18. https://doi.org/10.1186/s12978-019-0729-2

Wertz, R. W., & Wertz, D. C. (1989). *Lying-in: A history of childbirth in America*. Yale University Press.

Whipple, B., Josimovich, J. B., & Komisaruk, B. R. (1990). Sensory thresholds during the antepartum, intrapartum and postpartum periods. *International Journal of Nursing Studies*, *27*(3), 213–221. https://doi.org/10.1016/0020-7489(90)90036-I

Whipple, B., & Komisaruk, B. R. (1985). Elevation of pain threshold by vaginal stimulation in women. *Pain*, *21*(4), 357–367. https://doi.org/10.1016/0304-3959(85)90164-2

Whipple, B., & Komisaruk, B. R. (1988). Analgesia produced in women by genital self-stimulation. *Journal of Sex Research*, *24*(1), 130–140. https://doi.org/10.1080/00224498809551403

Yadav, G., McNamara S., & Gunturu S. (2024, January). Trauma-Informed Therapy. [Updated 2024 Aug 16]. In *StatPearls [Internet]*. StatPearls Publishing. www.ncbi.nlm.nih.gov/books/NBK604200/

Yeung, J., & Pauls, R. N. (2016). Anatomy of the vulva and the female sexual response. *Obstetrics and Gynecology Clinics*, *43*(1), 27–44. https://doi.org/10.1016/j.ogc.2015.10.011

APPENDICES

APPENDIX A

The Birth Pleasure Study Methodology and Methods

Study Methods and Methodology

The Birth Pleasure Study was designed to document and learn about experiences of pleasure in birth, presumed by myself and my advisors to be a rare occurrence in the context of the United States. As such, this study privileged saturation over representativeness; therefore, reaching saturation through the qualitative phase of the study was held as primary. Two main reasons drove this decision. First, birth pleasure is a poorly understood phenomenon that requires conceptual exploration and clarification before quantitative analyses based on discrete variables would become appropriate. Second, intersectional feminist and research justice orientations emphasize centering marginalized experiences and voices, without erasing the researcher's own. This is best accomplished by basing any quantitative work on rich and nuanced qualitative work.

The recruitment efforts aimed to achieve thematic saturation for the topic of study: birth pleasure experiences (Fusch & Ness, 2015; Guest et al., 2006). I used stratified purposive sampling (Teddlie & Yu, 2007, p. 90). Recruitment efforts involved in-person conversations as well as online communications using email and social media, particularly Facebook and Instagram, among my personal networks, organizational contacts, and listservs, locally (San Francisco Bay Area, Northern California) and on nonlocal platforms (online). The study design, recruitment materials and messaging, and informed consent forms were approved by the Human Research Review Committee at the California Institute of Integral Studies.

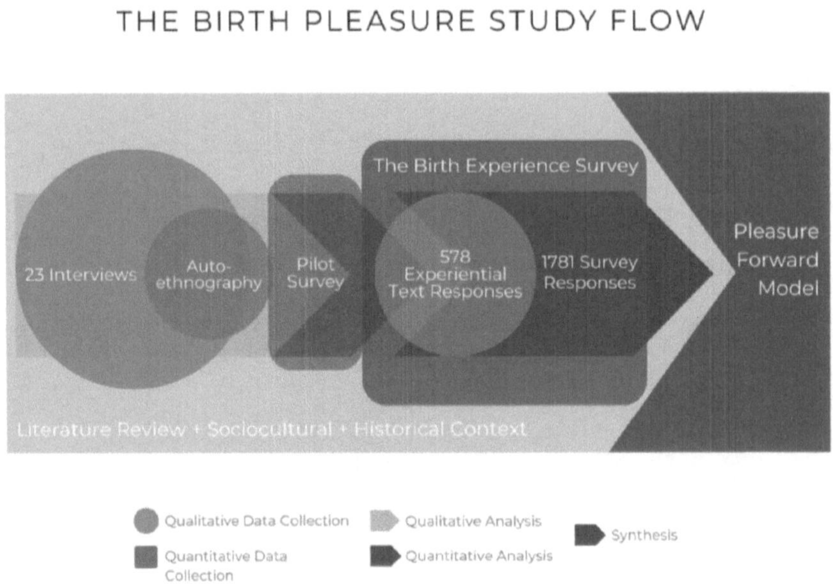

FIGURE A.1 Birth Pleasure Study Flow Chart.

A total of 41 people expressed interest in response to my study recruitment efforts. I contacted all 41 to schedule screens via the same method in which they indicated interest (typically email or social media message). Eleven did not respond to those messages to schedule the screening call. Potential participants were screened via phone call for eligibility.

A total of 28 people were screened, and all 28 were invited to participate in the study. Five did not respond to communications to schedule their interviews. One interested person was not invited to participate in a screening call due to known exclusionary severe mental health issues precluding ethical consent. In sum, 23 interviews were conducted.

Qualitative Phase: Semistructured Interviews

I conducted 23 interviews between May 2019 and February 2021: 21 were held online using the video-conferencing platform Zoom (due to both distance and to the COVID-19 pandemic) and two local interviews were held in-person, recorded using the Voice Memo Apple application. The interviews ranged in duration from roughly one to three hours and covered a total of 43 distinct birth experiences. I also conducted post-interview questionnaires to capture demographic data that did not emerge in the interviews.

Inclusion/Exclusion Criteria

Inclusion criteria included English-speaking (due to my own language limitations) birthing people, 18 years of age and older, who had given birth at least once, and had experienced pleasure (broadly defined) during the birth process. Exclusion criteria included those who had scheduled cesarean births with no trial of labor and those whose participation would be unethical (incapable of providing informed consent). Geographical location, duration of time since birth experience, or health status, including postpartum depression, anxiety, or posttraumatic stress disorder were not considered bases for exclusion. Out of a concern that the experience of pleasure during childbirth may be exceedingly rare, and in the absence of sufficient data to gauge this, it was deemed appropriate not to exclude participants based on when they had experienced birth pleasure or where.

Recruitment and Screening

With the goal of achieving thematic saturation (Fusch & Ness, 2015; Guest et al., 2006), I chose stratified purposive sampling (Teddlie & Yu, 2007, p. 90) through in-person conversations, online communications (mainly email and social media, particularly Facebook and Instagram). The primary wave of recruitment started with my close personal networks, and expanded into more distant organizational contacts (including health providers, health-related non-profit organizations, birthworker and doula collectives, professional practices including midwifery, physical therapy, and a number of other healing modalities that prioritize pregnant and birthing people. Eventually recruiting messages were distributed to various listservs, in my local area (namely the San Francisco Bay Area of Northern California) and then beyond as recruitment parameters were broadened to allow for participants nationwide and eventually outside US borders. Recruitment materials, including imagery and messaging, were approved by the Human Research Review Committee before dissemination.

Forty-one people responded to my study recruitment, all of whom were contacted to schedule screening conversations. Twenty-eight interested respondents were successfully screened via phone call and all were found eligible and invited to participate. Eleven did not respond to attempts to schedule the screening call.

Five invited participants did not respond to repeated attempts to schedule their interviews. Due to known exclusionary severe mental health issues precluding informed consent, one interested participant was not invited to screen. Ulitmately, I conducted 23 in-depth interviews. See Table A.1 for a summary of interview recruitment and participation.

TABLE A.1 Interview Recruitment Summary

n	*Recruitment status*
41	Total interested (responded to recruitment materials)
12	No response to schedule screening
1	Excluded prescreening (mental health issues precluding consent)
28	Screened
28	Eligible
5	No response to communications to schedule interview
23	Interviews completed (2 in-person, 21 via Zoom)

As Dána-Ain Davis (2019) has highlighted in her work on prematurity and obstetric racism, deep ethnographic work need not be tied to a shared geolocation but can be centered on a shared experience or concern for a specific issue. In this case, the shared experience was birth, an experience that spans the globe. Due to COVID-19 restrictions regarding in-person contact, as well as proximity and feasibility, most interviews took place via Zoom teleconference. Participant location was not limited. Zoom interviews typically took place in participants' homes, often with a baby bouncing on one knee. Traditional place-based ethnographic field notes on the lifestyles and living spaces were replaced with notes on the feel and tone of the site of the interview as experienced via Zoom. I did not collect qualitative data on neighborhood environs other than what was shared by participants directly.

There were some barriers to participation. Mothers/parents with young children may have had difficulty participating. Again, I conducted most interviews via Zoom teleconference, making the setting the choice of the participants. However, technological barriers may have been prohibitive for some who lacked a quality internet connection or an acceptable device for the Zoom application. Private and confidential settings were established for video conference interviews for both parties, and a discussion of this was a key part of scheduling and set-up. As the interviewer, I was in a private and closed space for all video conference interviews. The two in-person interviews were held in the participants' homes, the locations of their choosing. Both took place in Oakland, California, before the onset of the COVID-19 pandemic. See Table A.2 for a breakdown of participant location. With 23 interviews in total, I surpassed my recruitment goal of 20 interviews. Together, these 23 interviews covered a total of 43 distinct birth experiences. The average number of births per participant was 1.87 (1–5), and the mean time elapsed since birth at the time of the interview was 6.63 years (2 months–36 years; see Table A.3 and Figure A.2 below).

TABLE A.2 Geographic Location Breakdown: Interview Participants

Location		*Screened*	*Interviewed*
California	CA	11	9
New York	NY	4	4
Indiana	IN	2	2
Illinois	IL	1	1
Colorado	CO	1	1
Maryland	MD	1	1
Oregon	OR	1	1
Utah	UT	1	1
Wisconsin	WI	1	1
Florida	FL	1	0
Georgia	GA	1	0
England	UK	1	1
Israel	IL	1	1
Saskatchewan, Canada	SK	1	0
Total		**28**	**23**

TABLE A.3 Interview Data: Overview

	Total births	%	*Pleasurable*	%
Total births discussed in interviews	43	100	31	72
Hospital	24	56	13	54
Freestanding birth center	4	9	4	100
Home	15	35	14	93
Parity (births/participant)	$\bar{x}$ = 1.87 (1–5 births)			
Time since last birth @ interview	$\bar{x}$ = 6.63 years (2 months–36 years)			

I set out to attend to the gaps in the birth pleasure literature, with special regard to disparities in participation across racial/ethnic identity and socioeconomic position. Though I was unsuccessful in recruiting Native American/Indigenous (NAI) or Middle Eastern/North African (MENA) interview participants, I did largely achieve my goals of interviewing Black/African American, Latina/e/x, Asian/Pacific Islander (API), and Mixed-race participants (12 total) in equal or greater numbers than White participants (11), for 52.2% participation of people of color. Lower-socioeconomic status participants made up 39.1% of interviews, falling short of my goal

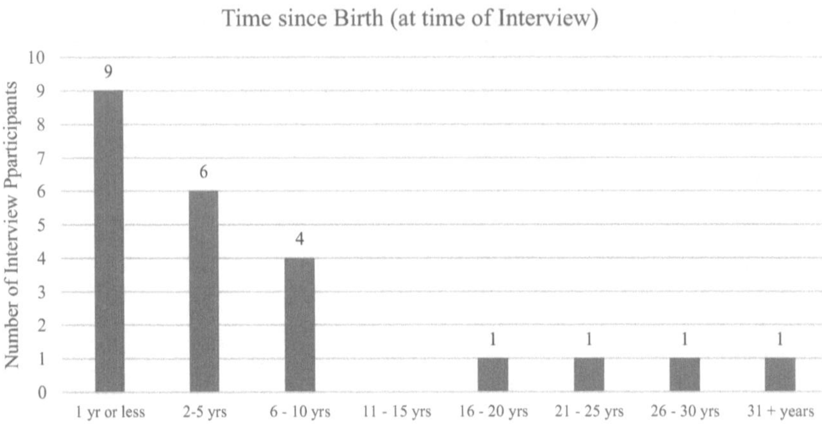

FIGURE A.2 Time Since Last Birth Experience at Time of Interview Across Participants.

TABLE A.4 Interview Participation: Participant Compared to Recruitment Goals

Race/ethnicity	*High income*		*Low income*		*Total*	
	N	*Goal*	*N*	*Goal*	*n*	*Goal*
API	3	2	0	2	3	4
Black (B)	2	2	3	2	5	4
Latina/e/x (L)	2	2	0	2	2	2
MENA (M)	0	1	0	1	0	1
NAI	0	1	0	1	0	1
Mixed Race	1 (B+L)	1	1 (W+M)	1	2	2
White (W)	6	2	5	2	11	4
Total	14	11	9	11	23	20

of 50%. See Table A.4 for more details on the study's recruitment goals and participation based on race/ethnicity and income.

Sexual and gender identity are rarely addressed in birth research. Often studies do not think to ask about the genders or sexual orientations of their participants, who are presumed cisgender and heterosexual at the outset due to cisheteronormative bias. I worked hard to include birthing people across a variety of gender expressions and sexualities in this study. In all, gender expansive people made up 13% of interview participants, and folks with nonheteronormative sexualities made up 26% of the interviews. Please see Table A.5 and Table A.6 for a breakdown of interview participation by sexual orientation and gender, and Table A.7 for a summary of the inclusivity of the study across several important points.

TABLE A.5 Interview Participants: Sexual Orientation Breakdown

Sexual orientation	*n*	%
Not exclusively heterosexual	6	26
Mostly heterosexual	1	4
Queer	1	4
Bisexual	3	13
Lesbian	1	4
Heterosexual	17	74

TABLE A.6 Interview Participants: Gender Identity Breakdown

Gender identity	*n*	%
Gender expansive	3	13
Agender/genderless	1	4
Nonbinary	1	4
Womxn	1	4
Cisgender women	20	87

TABLE A.7 Interview Participants: Overall Inclusion Summary

Participation inclusion	*Ratio*	%
People of color: White people	12: 11	52
Low income: Higher income	9: 14	39
Not exclusively heterosexual: Heterosexual	6: 11	26
Gender expansive: Cis-women	3: 20	13
Interviewees in California: Beyond California	9: 14	39
Screened in California: Beyond California	11: 17	39

Interview Protocols

First, the informed consent form included explanations of the risks, potential benefits, details of the interview process, and the pilot testing portion of the study. The informed consent process also included a review and discussion of the study procedures before starting the interview, where time was set aside for answering questions, addressing concerns, and emphasizing that participation is voluntary and can be stopped at any time. All consent forms were signed electronically as PDFs and received via email before the interview. Participants were asked in the consent form as well as verbally about their willingness to pilot test the survey. By email, I also secured an affirmation of continued consent before sending the pilot survey link to willing participants.

In a semistructured ethnographic interview format, I explored the study topic of birth pleasure experience with consenting participants. Twenty-one interviews were conducted via video- and audio-recorded Zoom teleconference and the two in-person interviews were audio-recorded. Most interviews ran roughly 90 minutes, except for one interview that went over two hours, with the participant's enthusiastic verbal consent to continue throughout (Kvale, 1996, pp. 124–159). I used introducing questions, follow-ups, probes, and clarifying questions (Kvale, 1996, pp. 133–135) in a flexible format to allow the participant to focus on those aspects of the topic that were most important to them (Kvale & Brinkmann, 2009), while staying on topic in the interview. The interview itself is a co-conducted intersubjective social interaction exploring the topic, and it is important to recognize that though the interview does collect data per se, it also co-creates it (Kvale, 1996, pp. 183–184).

APPENDIX B

Interview Participants: Snapshot

Pseudonym	*Key Identities and Demographics*	*Birth Experience Snapshot*
Aleks	White Russian-Armenian from Azerbaijan, Lesbian, Agender, married (open), post-college education (doctorate), high-income, living in Ijamsville, Maryland.	Pleasurable and pain-free births (in part) in de-medicalized third birth (first out-of-hospital), at a birth center, age 29, and de-medicalized fourth birth (second out-of-hospital) at home, age 36. Previous hospital births involved coerced cesareans, birth trauma, ages 22 and 25
Araceli	Mexican-American Latina from Mexico, heterosexual, cisgender woman, high-income, post-college education (masters) living in Oakland, California.	Pleasurable and pain-free (in part) de-medicalized second birth in hospital, age 39. Previous hospital birth not pleasurable, birth trauma, age 36
Bree	Vietnamese, from Vietnam, heterosexual, cisgender woman, married, with some college education, high-income, living in Saint George, Utah.	Pleasurable and pain-free (in full) first-and-only birth, at home, age 25

(*Continued*)

TABLE A.5 (Continued)

Pseudonym	*Key Identities and Demographics*	*Birth Experience Snapshot*
Callie	Black/African-American from Southern California, heterosexual, cisgender woman, married, high-income, post-college education (doctorate), living in Brooklyn, New York.	Pleasurable but not pain-free first-and-only birth, medicalized, induced due to hypertension and suspected pre-eclampsia, in hospital, age 42
Callisto	Black/African-American from Syracuse, New York, heterosexual, cisgender woman, married, post-college education (masters), high-income, living in Urbana, Illinois.	Pleasurable and pain-free (except a tear at delivery) first-and-only birth, at home, age 27
Cande	Latine Mestize from Santa Barbara, California, Non-binary Queer, married, post-college education (doctorate), high-income, living in Red Hook, New York.	Pleasurable and pain-free (minus moments of confinement: car ride or fetal monitoring, also coccyx injury at delivery) first-and-only birth, at a birth center, age 36
Chandra	Black (African-American, Afro-Caribbean, Afro-Panamanian) from Brooklyn New York, heterosexual, cisgender woman, married (first birth), partnered (second birth), middle-income, post-college education (masters), living in Oakland, California.	Pleasurable and pain-free first (twin) and second (singleton) births, in hospital, ages 19 and 23 (first birth entirely pain-free minus fight with nurse)
Dalisay	Filipina from the Philippines, heterosexual, cisgender woman, married, high-income, post-college education (masters), living in Alameda, California.	Pleasurable and painful first and second births, medicalized, in hospital setting, at ages 31 and 43

TABLE A.5 (Continued)

Pseudonym	*Key Identities and Demographics*	*Birth Experience Snapshot*
Debbie	White, heterosexual, cisgender woman, married, post-college education (doctorate), of middle-high-income, living in Colorado.	Pleasurable and painful first and second births, medicalized, in hospital setting, at ages 20 and 32
Fabia	Spanish, from Spain, white, mostly heterosexual, cisgender woman, married, post-college education (masters), high-income, living in Thrapston, England.	Second birth, at home, unattended free birth, age 35, previous unattended free birth at home at age 33 not referred to as pleasurable
Malika	Black/African-American, heterosexual, cisgender woman, married, low-income, with bachelors-level education, unhoused, with public health insurance.	First-and-only birth, a birth-center transfer (due to meconium) to a hospital where she received an epidural and pitocin augmentation, and ultimately delivered vaginally, age 39
Marion	White (Dutch) from Calistoga, California, heterosexual, cisgender woman, married, low-middle-income, with some college education, living in Dunsmuir, California.	Pleasurable and Pain-free Second birth (first out-of-hospital) VBAC at a birth center, age 23 (some cervical pinching, and fear-associated pain with the last bit of stretch at delivery). First birth in hospital, cesarean, birth trauma, not pleasurable, age 21
Melissa	Black/African-American and Latina mixed from New York, heterosexual, cisgender woman, married, high-income, with some college education, living in Brooklyn, New York.	Pleasurable but painful second birth (first out-of-hospital birth) at home, age 32; Previous hospital birth age 19 not considered pleasurable
Nava	White Israeli Jew, from New York, heterosexual, cisgender woman, married, low-income, post-college education (masters), living in Moshav Sharona, Israel.	Pleasurable and pain-free (minus the car ride) first-and-only birth, precipitous, in a birth center, age 28

(*Continued*)

TABLE A.5 (Continued)

Pseudonym	*Key Identities and Demographics*	*Birth Experience Snapshot*
Pearl	White, from Massachusetts, bisexual, cisgender woman, married, low-middle-income, post-college education (masters), living in Oregon.	Pleasurable but not pain-free first-and-only birth, at home, age 30
Raquel	Chinese, from Washington state, heterosexual, cisgender woman, married, high-income, post-college education (masters), living in San Francisco, California.	Pleasurable, pain-free (minus very intense pitocin contractions at transition, just before epidural was placed) first-and-only birth, induction without anesthesia for most of labor, at a hospital, age 37
Romi	White-passing Moroccan Jew, heterosexual, cisgender woman, married, high-income, post-college education (masters), living in Oakland, California.	Pleasurable and painful first and second births, both medicalized, in hospital setting, at ages 31 and 33
Sankofa	Black/African-American from New York, bisexual, cisgender woman, married, high-income, post-college education (doctorate), living in Yonkers, New York.	Pleasurable but not pain-free births in de-medicalized third, fourth, and fifth births at home, ages 28, 30, and 36; Previous hospital births involved birth mistreatment, ages 23 and 26
Semiramis	Arab+European mixed, single, queer womxn, from Massachusetts, low-income, educated (masters), living in Berkeley, California.	Pleasurable but not pain-free first-and-only birth, at hospital, age 22
Skylar	White, heterosexual, cisgender woman, married, low-middle-income, high-school level educated, living in West DeMoines, Iowa.	Pleasurable and pain-free second birth (first out-of-hospital), at home, age 24

TABLE A.5 (Continued)

Pseudonym	*Key Identities and Demographics*	*Birth Experience Snapshot*
Theia	White, lesbian, cisgender woman, married to a man at the time of the birth, low-income, with some college education, living in Au Claire, Wisconsin.	Third birth (first out-of-hospital), at home, age 29
Venus	White, from San Diego, California, heterosexual (previously bisexual) cisgender woman, married, high-income, post-college education (masters), living in Northern California.	Pleasurable but not pain-free first and second births, at home, age 28 and 31
Veronica	White, born in Okinawa Japan to military family, heterosexual cisgender woman, married, low-middle-income, post-college education (masters), living in Iowa.	Pleasurable but not pain-free first birth at hospital, age 33 and second birth at home age 36

APPENDIX C

Interview Participant Demographics Tables

TABLE A.8 Interview Participant Location and Demographics: Race, Ethnic Identity, Place of Origin

		Race, Ethnic Identity, Place of Origin	
Pseudonym	*Location*	*Race/Ethnicity*	*Origin*
Aleks	MD	White Russian-Armenian	Azerbaijan
Araceli	CA	Latina Mexican-American Binational	Mexico City, MX
Bree	UT	Asian/Pacific Islander Vietnamese	Vietnam
Callie	NY	Black/African American	Harbor City, CA
Callisto	IL	Black/African American	Syracuse, NY
Cande	NY	Latine Mexican Mestize	Santa Barbara, CA
Chandra	CA	Black/African American	Brooklyn, NY
Dalisay	CA	Asian/Pacific Islander Filipina	Philippines
Debbie	CO	White	Unstated
Fabia	England	White Spaniard	Avila, Spain
Malika	CA	Black/African American	Berkeley, CA
Marion	CA	White Dutch	Calistoga, CA
Melissa	NY	Black/African American + Latina	Brooklyn, NY
Nava	Israel	White Ashkenazi Israeli Jew	White Plains, NY
Pearl	OR	White	Worcester, MA
Raquel	CA	Asian/Pacific Islander Chinese	Washington state
Romi	CA	White-passing Moroccan Jew	Oakland, CA

TABLE A.8 (Continued)

		Race, Ethnic Identity, Place of Origin	
Sankofa	NY	Black/African American	Yonkers, NY
Semiramis	CA	Arab + European	Melrose, MA
Skylar	IA	White	Unstated
Theia	WI	White	Eau Claire, WI
Venus	CA	White	San Diego, CA
Veronica	IA	White	Okinawa, Japan

Note: Location abbreviations refer to states in the United States only.

TABLE A.9 Interview Participant Demographics: Sexuality, Gender, and Relationship Status

	Sexuality, Gender, and Relationship		
Pseudonym	*Gender*	*Sexual Orientation*	*Relationship Status*
Aleks	Agender Queer	L	Married Open
Araceli	Cis/Woman	H	Married Exclusive
Bree	Cis/Woman	H	Married Exclusive
Callie	Cis/Woman	H	Married Exclusive
Callisto	Cis/Woman	H	Married Exclusive
Cande	Non-binary	Q	Married Exclusive
Chandra	Cis/Woman	H	Single
Dalisay	Cis/Woman	H	Married Exclusive
Debbie	Cis/Woman	H	Married Exclusive
Fabia	Cis/Woman	Hm	Married Exclusive
Malika	Cis/Woman	H	Married Exclusive
Marion	Cis/Woman	H	Married Exclusive
Melissa	Cis/Woman	H	Married Exclusive
Nava	Cis/Woman	H	Married Exclusive
Pearl	Cis/Woman	Bi	Married Exclusive
Raquel	Cis/Woman	H	Married Exclusive
Romi	Cis/Woman	H	Married Exclusive
Sankofa	Cis/Woman	Bi	Married Open
Semiramis	Womxn	Q	Single
Skylar	Cis/Woman	H	Married Exclusive
Theia	Cis/Woman	L	Single
Venus	Cis/Woman	H/Bi (prior)	Married Exclusive
Veronica	Cis/Woman	H	Married Exclusive

Note: Sexual orientation abbreviations refer to participants' self-described identities as follows: L (lesbian), Bi (bisexual), Q (queer), H (heterosexual), Hm (heterosexual mostly). Abbreviations used in this and following charts are summarized in Table A.12.

TABLE A.10 Interview Participant Demographics: Socioeconomic Status and Class Factors

Pseudonym	*Socioeconomic Status and Class Factors*					
	Annual Income US$	*Family Size*	*Housing*	*Occupation*	*Insurance*	*Education*
Aleks	$90,000	6	Own	Professor, author	P/EB	6
Araceli	$90,000	4	Rent	Educational researcher	P/EB	6
Bree	$100,000	3	Rent	Business partner	None	4
Callie	$200,000	3	Rent	Public health, academic	P/EB	6
Callisto	$90,000	3	Own	Doula	P/EB	6
Cande	$106,000	3	Own	Consultant and Researcher	P/EB	6
Chandra	$64,000	3	Own	Doula, Doula educator	P/EB	6
Dalisay	$250,000	4	Own	Government	P/EB	6
Debbie	Med-High*	4	Own	Teaching/Nursing	P/EB	6
Fabia	$99,000	4	Own	Midwife	Public	5
Malika	$20,000	3	Unhoused	Poet	Public	5
Marion	$55,000	4	Rent	Stay-at-home mother	P/EB	4
Melissa	$120,000	4	Rent/Own	Doula	P/EB	4
Nava	$18,000	3	Rent/Own	Student Creative Writing	Public	6
Pearl	$38,000	3	Own	Acad. admin, counselor	Public	6
Raquel	$300,000	3	Rent	Designer	P/EB	6
Romi	$100,000	4	Own	Therapist	P/EB	6
Sankofa	$60,000	7	Own	Midwife	P/EB	6

Semiramis	$25,000	2	Rent	Massage therapist, doula	P/EB	6
Skylar	$60,000	4	Rent	Stay-at-home mother	None	3
Theia	$20,000	4	Rent	Midwifery student	Public	4
Venus	$150,000	4	Own	Therapist	P/EB	6
Veronica	$45,000	4	Own	Midwife	P/EB	6

Note: Abbreviations used here Abbreviations and numerical education levels used in this chart are summarized in Table A.12. P/EB refers to Private/Employment-based health insurance coverage.

* This participant declined to state a figure but reported medium to high range of income.

TABLE A.11 Interview Participant Demographics: Spirituality and Religion

Pseudonym	*Spirituality and Religious Identity*
Aleks	Other – Atheist Witch
Araceli	Raised Catholic, now SbnR
Bree	SbnR
Callie	SbnR
Callisto	SbnR
Cande	Raised Catholic, now SbnR
Chandra	Catholic
Dalisay	SbnR
Debbie	Pagan
Fabia	SbnR
Malika	Christian (Non-denominational)
Marion	Christian (Non-denominational)
Melissa	SbnR
Nava	Jewish, Observant
Pearl	SbnR
Raquel	No religious beliefs
Romi	Jewish, Conservative
Sankofa	SbnR
Semiramis	Polytheistic
Skylar	Christian (Non-denominational)
Theia	Christian (Lutheran)
Venus	Interfaith
Veronica	Other – Secular Humanist

Note: Abbreviation SbnR denotes "spiritual but not religious" (one of the more common responses with regard to spiritual and religious identity).

TABLE A.12 Key of Abbreviations: Interview Participant Demographics

Demographic Factor	*Abbreviation*	*Meaning*
Sexual orientation	H	Heterosexual
	Hm	Mostly Heterosexual
	Bi	Bisexual
	Q	Queer
	L	Lesbian
Education	1	Elementary school (K–6th)
	2	Middle school (7–8th)
	3	High school/GED (9th–12th)
	4	Some college/Trade school (Associates, Trade certificate)
	5	College graduate (Bachelors)
	6	Post-college (Graduate school, Masters, Doctorate)
Insurance	P/EB	Private/Employer-Based
Spirituality/Religious Identity	SbnR	Spiritual but not Religious

INDEX

Note: Figures are indicated by *italics*. Tables are indicated by **bold**.